Intimacy

Intimacy

A field guide to finding connection
and feeling your deep desires

Ita O'Brien

with Sarah Crompton

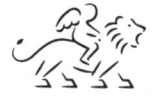

THE DIAL PRESS
NEW YORK

I dedicate this book to the power of zjumpness
to Russell, Zac, and Zoe

CONTENTS

CONTENTS

FOREWORD

BY GILLIAN ANDERSON

When I first encountered Ita O'Brien's work as an intimacy coordinator, it was on the set of *Sex Education*. As someone who has spent decades portraying myriad intimate relationships onscreen, I was struck by how her presence transformed what had historically been one of the most vulnerable and potentially problematic aspects of performance into something safe, empowering, and indeed collaborative.

The impact of Ita's work extends far beyond the entertainment industry. Her groundbreaking approach to intimacy—based on consent, clear communication, and respect—offers wisdom that can enrich all our relationships. Just as she helped me and countless other actors navigate intimate scenes with confidence and authenticity, this book provides a road map for exploring intimate relations in our everyday lives.

What makes this book extraordinary is how it reframes conversations about intimacy. Rather than focusing solely on the physical aspects of sexual relationships, Ita explores the full spectrum of human connection—from the first tentative glances between potential lovers to the deep bonds that sustain long-term partnerships. She shows us that true intimacy begins with understanding ourselves and learning to communicate our needs and boundaries clearly.

As an actor and as a woman, I've witnessed firsthand how cultural attitudes toward intimacy are evolving. Yet many of us still struggle to talk openly about our desires, fears, and needs. This book arrives at a crucial moment, offering practical guidance while celebrating the profound importance of intimate connection in all its forms.

And Ita's voice—wise, compassionate, and direct— guides us through this territory with remarkable sensitivity. A true gift to have out in the world.

HOW TO USE
THIS BOOK

Throughout my career, I have gathered, been inspired by, experienced, and integrated so many wonderful practitioners' wisdom and practice into the work I am sharing with you. Bonnie Bainbridge-Cohen, Gabrielle Roth, Betty Martin, and Jill Purce are a few who have touched me on my journey, but there have been many more.

Just as there is a joy in losing yourself to the music while dancing, there's a freedom and joy to be found in following your curiosity. So, if anything in this book inspires you, follow that inspiration and go learn more. I've included recommended resources at the end of the book to help you.

As we take the journey through the book, I will share exercises I often undertake with actors. I hope that they will help you to feel more grounded, connected, and present in your body and mind. Because this work is such a foundation of the intimacy journey, you will find more exercises at the beginning of the book, but each chapter also contains exercises and resources that can bring you closer to yourself, and closer to the people in your life.

My invitation is for you to read the exercises and then physically try them out. In the audiobook you can listen to me talk you through them.

Enjoy!

Intimacy

PROLOGUE

AN INTIMATE SCENE

A girl sits opposite a boy on a bed, twisting a cup nervously in her hand. They are around 17 years old. He sits on a chair, near but just out of reach, watching her intently. The air between them crackles.

Their conversation is quiet and revealing. She confesses that she feels like a misfit; he tells her that he doesn't know how he feels most of the time. "And what about now?" she asks. He doesn't answer, but instead stands, goes to her as she sits on the bed, and gently kisses her. She kisses him back. "Now can we take our clothes off?" she asks. He laughs. "Yeah, yeah," he answers with a smile.

They do, undressing each other slowly at first, then taking their own clothes off. He kisses her neck; he reaches out and gives her erotic pleasure; she touches him back, shyly exploring, giving him erotic pleasure. Then they move onto the bed. "Do you have a condom?" she asks. "Yeah . . ." he says, continuing, "Is that what you want?" He takes one from a shelf, but adds, "Are you sure this is what you want?" She nods. "If it hurts, I'll stop." He puts on the condom and then kisses her gently. She gasps as she registers penetration. He asks, "Does it hurt?" She replies, "A bit," as she looks up at him and smiles. "It's nice." And they tenderly make love.

Many of you will recognize this scene where Marianne and Connell make love for the first time, in the second episode of the BBC series adaptation of Sally Rooney's novel *Normal People*. It has had an extraordinary impact. The series, tracing the course of an affair between two Irish teenagers from different backgrounds, first shown in 2020, made stars of Daisy Edgar-Jones and Paul Mescal, who played the young lovers. Even the chain Mescal wore around his neck became a cult object on the internet.

It was a brilliant piece of storytelling, perfectly adapted for the screen by Rooney herself with Alice Birch and Mark O'Rowe and directed with sensitivity and nuance by Lenny Abrahamson and Hettie Macdonald. But it was something more than that. It was a depiction of intimacy that was both realistic and explicit. Its truthfulness resonated with audiences worldwide. In fact, it resonated so strongly with the viewer that, for many, it was the experience that introduced them to the very concept of an intimacy coordinator, and the idea that the intimacy we see on-screen can have a profound experience on our "real" lives.

I was the intimacy coordinator on *Normal People*, and because the sex scenes attracted so much attention, it was perhaps the first time that many people became aware of the role. My job involves helping the creative team to build a narrative of intimacy that is convincing, serving the director's vision, creating clear choreography so that the actors feel safe and empowered, and the sexual content is not gratuitous, but an essential part of the story.

From the moment I became involved in the production, it was clear that it was special, that I was part of something really exciting. I can't take any credit for the incredible writing that was already in the show, or Abrahamson's exceptional direction, the amazing acting by Paul Mescal and Daisy Edgar-Jones, or the way that the cinematographer, Suzie Lavelle, frames every scene. But I did have something to do with the way that lovemaking is depicted.

I think director Lenny Abrahamson put it very well when he told the Edinburgh TV Festival in August 2020: "One of the principles that we all shared . . . was to try not to distinguish the intimacy scenes from the rest of the drama and not to go into 'sex scene' mode. We wanted to make sure what we were doing in those scenes deepened the understanding of the characters and what was occurring between them."[1] In many ways, this is also the key to understanding intimacy in our own lives: we can't just switch to "sex scene" mode and expect to have good sex, but instead need to understand it as an extension of the connections we establish in our lives, both with ourselves and with others.

The intimate scenes between Marianne and Connell were also remarkable because the actors, Edgar-Jones and Mescal, found it creatively satisfying and ultimately rewarding. This was especially gratifying to me. Paul Mescal gave an interview afterward in which he said, "I felt totally safe and bolstered . . . because the process was so steadfast, you can really lean into the characters' passion for each other, because you're not worried about the physical blocking anymore."[2] That's exactly how it should be. But in another interview, he added something more: "The prospect of bringing something to the screen that I felt was representative of the reality of young people in love having sex was really exciting to me."

This statement is remarkable, but it shouldn't be. We're so used to watching screen depictions of intimacy where this isn't the case. They are devoid of real emotion. A couple meet and then it cuts to a sex scene, as if their physical relationship is separate from every other aspect of their lives. We've become accustomed to seeing portrayals of sex that are robotic, athletic, and gratuitous. It's rare to see the kind of relationships we've all experienced in real life: an expression of connection that is clumsy, awkward, funny, and—hopefully—ultimately satisfying.

The end result of approaching sex scenes in this way does not just develop into a great piece of television. If you watch it moment by moment, it can become the most beautiful embodiment of the best realities of our intimate lives: of the joy of connection, of the excitement of passion, of the way that consent can be sought and given without stopping sex being erotic and exciting. There is a beat in the scene that particularly affected viewers. At the moment of penetration, Connell is talking to Marianne, saying he will stop if she doesn't like it. He acknowledges that she is a virgin, letting her make the decisions about the nature of their encounter.

I am bowled over by how many people say watching this encounter has affected them, that it has helped them to remember all the joy and gorgeousness of their first relationships as teenagers, and how unsure they felt. Sally Rooney's writing truly captures the point of view of a young person, full of doubt about their feelings and a lack of confidence in who they are in the world. Things go wrong for Connell and Marianne later in the story, yet when they first have sex, they manage to look after each other perfectly, sharing in a clearly consensual experience that is a pleasure for them both. This radically fresh viewpoint in the way intimate connection is portrayed has won many awards, and even more fans. The fact that it has been shown in secondary schools in the UK, as a means of helping young people negotiate consent in their own relationships, is something of which I'm particularly proud.

On or off the screen, none of this is easy. You're not negotiating with a film crew in your bedroom, but if you want to find true intimacy, then you probably need to find a way of talking to your prospective sexual partner about what will satisfy you and what you do and don't want to do. It can be hard to know how to express our desires to a partner. It can be even harder to know what we actually want, or what our bodies are telling us. When we embark on intimate relationships, it can be challenging to set our boundaries. But if you think about what you want and what you are into, then you are taking responsibility for your desires. It is then possible to make your intentions clear, to have a conversation with your partner, negotiating what you want from a sexual encounter. In the throes of sex, it can be particularly difficult to say something suddenly, to put a boundary in place.

To release into the joy and pleasure of connection, it would help to be supported by a field guide to intimacy— not just onscreen but in our lives. Just as the Intimacy on Set Guidelines I use in the workplace offer a process of open communication, consent, choreography, and closure in the creation of intimate scenes onscreen, so too could a field guide to intimacy support in our lives. My expertise has led me to the point where I can help create a sex scene as a body dance where everybody is empowered, and everyone feels safe. But it's more than that. Safety, agreement, and consent are interwoven with that concept; but it's also about portraying intimacy in ways that are beautiful and believable. I don't want intimate scenes to be less sexy. If anything, I want them to have more plausible, sensual, sexual, erotic, and emotional truth, to bring them closer to our lived experiences.

I don't know everything about intimacy. I am not a sex therapist, a counselor, or a healer. They all have their specialized fields. I have mine. Not all the skills I have developed can transfer to life. I can't walk into someone's bedroom and choreograph their sexual intercourse. (Even though I have actually been asked to do that!) But I can help you understand, and work toward, some of the conditions that I've found are essential to creating an environment in which intimacy can take seed, grow, and thrive.

Just as my work onscreen has been like a pebble thrown in a pond, creating ripples that have affected how the entertainment industry depicts sexual encounters, I hope this book will open up those conversations in individual lives that will help to create a more truthful and authentic attitude to yourself and your relationships with your partners. I also hope the techniques I share with you in this book can support you to make healthier and more genuine connections, whether it be with your families, your friends, or your romantic partners. Drawing on what I have learned in staging intimate content, I am going to suggest some ways of deepening intimacy that you can apply to your life.

In this context, it's important to remember that according to its dictionary definition, intimacy is a close familiarity or friendship. Only euphemistically has it come to mean sexual intercourse. Sex can be an outcome of intimacy, but it is only part of the definition of the word. People think intimacy is about another person, but, for me, it is first and foremost about understanding ourselves. I sometimes imagine breaking the word down: "into me see" and that journey of loving, accepting, and respecting yourself. Then you can take that into your relationship with someone else.

If we learn to listen to our bodies as well as our minds, to recognize and express our own needs and desires, to have the courage and the understanding to articulate our boundaries, and to respect those of our sexual and intimate partners, then I hope we can work toward enriching our relationships and experiences of pleasure, leading to fuller, more authentic lives: a utopia where society is shaped around communication and authentic connection.

What I am outlining is a new language of intimacy. This is my field guide to finding connection and a way of fulfilling our deepest desires.

CHAPTER ONE

THE MIRROR

WHY WHAT WE SEE ONSCREEN MATTERS

Making realistic art matters. When Shakespeare's Hamlet tells the troupe of players that they need to hold a mirror up to nature, he is describing the role that theater, books, and films have had in our lives since time immemorial. Art looks at the dilemmas that humankind faces and invites us to see ourselves.

As an increasingly screen-based society, our screens (and our stages) become a reflecting glass. If the intimate content we see is unrealistic, separated from its emotional narrative, then it is telling us a lie about ourselves. It's making us less honest, less open. It is in danger of making us behave in ways that are destructive to ourselves and our relationships. If what we see is complex, truthful, and challenging, then the entertainment industry can help society understand itself better.

People are often turned off by the sex they see onscreen, not because it is explicit but because it isn't real. All that bumping and grinding, the thrusting and heads thrown back in simulated ecstasy rarely bears much relationship to people's own experience of their sexual encounters. Yet, if you think back to the films you watched when you were growing up, then you might notice that they have conditioned what you now expect in your intimate life.

In explicit sexual scenes, we nearly always see spontaneous penetration after perhaps 30 seconds of kissing. Is that how it happens in your life? No! Certainly not for anyone I know. Men take time to get erect; women need to open like a flower and certainly some form of lubrication. You might argue that it doesn't matter, that what we see onscreen is fiction and it doesn't affect what happens in real life. But it does.

First-time lovemaking and the loss of virginity is nearly always glamorized, as in *Gossip Girl,* or romanticized, as in *The Notebook*. The reason the scene between Connell and Marianne in *Normal People* hit home so strongly is because that type of naturalism is so rare. It comes so much closer to many people's first experience of sex, yet it isn't depicted that way onscreen.

These media portrayals matter. Productions can set a tone for a whole cultural moment. If you happened to be going to cinemas in the 1990s, there was an entire genre of hugely popular films in which women were essentially bought. The charm of Julia Roberts's performance in *Pretty Woman* disguised the fact that she was a sex worker being paid for her time by a rich man. The box-office charisma of Robert Redford somehow made the premise of *Indecent Proposal*—that it was OK for a man to offer a stranger a million dollars for a night with his wife—acceptable.

Onscreen, women are often depicted as being cajoled into sex, as if that is a normal way to behave, or enjoying sex after it has been forced upon them, which goes beyond abnormal into dangerous. They are rarely depicted as initiating sex, which creates the illusion that men always need to draw them into a sexual encounter for sex to happen.

But the issue is greater than individual films. Because the people literally calling the shots as the directors and cinematographers are mostly men (and it's worth noting that as of 2025, it was still the case that a woman hadn't won the Best Cinematography Oscar), a subsection of the population has shaped how the whole of society views women, men, and the sexual relations between them. Hollywood has gendered the shot design of films, so that women and men are consistently portrayed differently onscreen.

The feminist filmmaker Nina Menkes explores this brilliantly in her film documentary *Brainwashed: Sex-Camera-Power.*[1] At its simplest, the shot design of most films perpetuates the notion that women are passive creatures, longing to be looked at, whereas men are invariably in positions of power. Women are often shot two-dimensionally, surrounded by ethereal lighting, not anchored in the environment but somehow floating in some ageless netherworld. There is no sense of a woman being grounded in reality in many films. The men, in contrast, are shown in full, rounded 3-D. It doesn't matter if the result is a great film or a pile of shlock, the basic grammar of cinema is reinforcing the sense that women are objects of desire, sitting or lying around and looking beautiful, while men are active beings, always ready to do something.

I was on the set of a film where the scene was meant to be one where the woman, as protagonist, told her husband something of vital importance. Yet the director—unconsciously, I think—put the woman in profile while the husband was full face on. I was watching the filming on the monitor, sitting next to the female writer of the script. She kept saying, under her breath, "Make her the protagonist." Yet the director seemed entirely unaware of what he was doing. The scene had been written to show the woman's point of view; it was shot to reflect the man's.

This conscious or unconscious viewpoint permeates the fabric of our thinking. It is the default glass through which we see the world. When I was doing my MA in Movement Studies, one of our tutors shared an exercise with us as students in which we explored the fundamental mindset of masculine and feminine. A chair was set in the center of the room, and we were asked to walk in and sit in it. When we were in a masculine mode, the entire thought pattern was about taking up space, looking for where the exits were, weighing up the dangers. The body language revealed someone powerful and in charge.

For the feminine mindset, we were to walk in and arrange ourselves, shaping our body into beautiful curves, diagonal lines, ready to be looked at, to receive admiration and incite desire. This always enraged me; I never saw why I should accept that this helplessness was a natural quality of being womanly. Nevertheless, for an actor, it is a truthful reflection of how women are seen and quite often how they behave in film and TV scripts.

The trouble is that the screen image of a dominant man and a submissive woman reinforces and creates inequalities. It limits our ability to see ourselves and each other occupying spaces outside of those roles. Beyond that, the rise of the erotic thriller and Hollywood's glamorization of sexual assault has had a chilling effect offscreen. It both reflects what is happening in the real world and also suggests it is normal. All of which means that we have to be serious and careful when it comes to intimate content.

Since the start of storytelling onscreen, intimate content has been treated as an improvisation exercise, one where actors are simply required to get on with it. Actors would never be asked to make up a fight scene, because they weren't experienced fight directors, or to choreograph a tango when they knew nothing about dance. Yet they'd consistently been asked to make up sex scenes because it's assumed we all know what to do when it comes to sex. That has led to abuse and trauma. It has damaged actors' creativity and their ability to perform, and indeed is still occurring. In May 2024, Denise Gough, who won an Olivier award for her role in *People, Places and Things*, called on those in positions of power in the industry to become "allies for colleagues" and noted that we are in "an industry where misconduct remains rife."[2]

All too often, before I created the Intimacy on Set Guidelines (which I will talk about later) to formalize best practices in the industry when working with scenes involving intimacy, simulated sex, and nudity, a kind of chaos reigned.

In recent times, some of the most prolonged and extensive sex scenes that have been televised came in the sensationally popular *Game of Thrones.* Yet, Gemma Whelan, one of the stars, described the multiple intimate scenes as a "frenzied mess." "They used to say, when we shout action, just go for it . . . A director might say, 'Bit of boob biting, then slap her bum and go . . .' "[3] What seems "sexy" onscreen can feel anything but for the people involved.

On June 6, 2021, the actor and writer Michaela Coel made a speech that drew attention to the difference that intimacy coordination can make, as she collected a BAFTA award for best actress for her groundbreaking series *I May Destroy You*. Out of the blue, and to my great astonishment and pride, she dedicated the award to me.

> Thank you for your existence in our industry, for making the space safe, for creating physical, emotional, and professional boundaries so that we can make work about exploitation, loss of respect, about abuse of power, without being exploited or abused in the process. I know what it is like to shoot without an intimacy director—the messy, embarrassing feeling for the crew, the internal devastation for the actor. Your direction was essential to my show, and I believe essential for every production company that wants to make work exploring themes of consent.[4]

It was one of the most cherished moments in my career, but it was also an important milestone on the road to the recognition of the intimacy practitioner's vital role. It drew attention to the fact that the problem with sex in filmmaking was essentially the same as the problem with sex in real life: people were too embarrassed to talk about it. In the face of that embarrassment, intimate content becomes the elephant in the room, and in that silent space, a lot of bad practice occurs. "The internal devastation for the actor" that Michaela described was a sensation that so many women—and quite a few men—had felt not just on set but also in their private lives.

It begins with a sense of awkwardness when we are asked to do something that makes us feel uncomfortable. We go along with it because we don't want to make a fuss. Our chest tightens, but we put on a brave smile and carry on. Or we are coerced into something. When you try to push back, you are told it's not a big deal. Perhaps you override your instincts for the sake of a simple life and for fear of causing a scene. Disregarding your feelings can lead to escalation from feeling uncomfortable, to feeling harassed or to feeling absolutely abused.

Until very recently, in the entertainment industry, this emotional and psychological injury hadn't been acknowledged, described, or spoken much about. The wreckage has taken different forms for different people. It might have been a knot in the stomach someone felt when they were sent a script and realized that there was a sex scene and nudity and decided to walk away from a role they really wanted because they weren't comfortable exposing themselves in that way. It might have been the shocking moment in an audition when someone was asked to kiss multiple people to test out their sexual compatibility, as if a real-life attraction can ever be substituted for a performance. It might be the chaos that actors describe when they are asked by a director simply to "go for it," trying to negotiate a professional way through the creation of the most intimate scenes.

My journey into the work I now do began in 2014 with the desire to devise a play, *Does My Sex Offend You?*, exploring the dynamic of the perpetrator and the victim. We started the process toward its eventual staging by exploring catcalling on the street, which had potency for everybody in the room, men and women alike. The experience of the invasion of your space, the entitlement of the caller who thinks you should be grateful for a wolf whistle or a shouted remark, the impact on the body of being objectified resonated with everyone. Responses varied from feeling unsafe to wanting to disappear, to feeling the need to push back with a false bravado.

In exploring these incidents with the actors, I was astonished at the seriousness of the impact on the participants' lives, men and women alike. We tend to write off such behavior as normal, but in fact it is the background noise to much more serious incidents of harassment, abuse, and even assault. In response to this sense of permanent hostility, in 2012, the former actor Laura Bates founded The Everyday Sexism Project to record instances of sexism "experienced on a day-to-day basis, serious and minor, outrageously offensive or so niggling and normalized that you don't even feel able to protest."[5]

In *Everyday Sexism*, her subsequent book, Bates wrote:

> People who shout at women in the street don't do it because they think there's a chance the woman will drop her shopping, willy-nilly, and leap into their arms! It isn't a compliment—and to call it that disparages the vast majority of lovely men who are perfectly able to pay a real compliment. It's an exertion of power, dominance and control, and it's utterly horrifying that we've become so used to it that it's considered the norm.[6]

I admire the Everyday Sexism campaign. It feels part of the arc I have lived through where society is more sensitive to calling out bad behavior and demanding we behave better.

Although I can still see so much that needs to be done, when I look back on my career, I can also appreciate that attitudes have improved.

My own journey reflects the mood. My parents came from rural Ireland, at a time when the Catholic Church still dominated the way that people lived and where sex—and particularly sexual abuse—was hidden away, never to be discussed or acknowledged. When I was 14, I was told by my mother that if I ever lived with my boyfriend, my family would disown me. Such strictures have all but vanished.

In my career, too, I started out as a dancer, training from the age of 3 in ballet, and from 16 onward including musical theater, working professionally from the age of 18. In the 1980s, assumptions about dancers in the industry—and by my dad!—were not so different from those that had dogged dance as a professional career since the nineteenth century. Essentially, dancers were there to be at the beck and call of powerful men who did not respect them.

Sometimes the demands were quite explicit: my first job in a dance group touring Asia required me to dance topless in four out of the fourteen numbers. Later, when I auditioned to be a body double for a leading actress, we were lined up in our bikinis. I was chosen to portray the actress's upper body, dancing topless. I was flattered but knew that I wouldn't feel comfortable, and so I turned it down. I decided not even to audition for an advertisement for a famous perfume brand, to be filmed in black and white, with the camera panning along the shore of the sea and boulders and rocks, and then panning along the naked back of a woman. I could see how tastefully this was intended to be shot, but said to my agent that I knew I would not feel comfortable with being fully naked.

It wasn't just in front of the camera that there were choices to be made. I was one of the pantomime chorus dancers where the star, a household name at the time, told the women in the chorus that he expected someone to service his sexual demands. If you wanted not to be harassed, you got good at vanishing quickly at the end of parties, never letting anyone take you home. A producer told me that he had watched me over the years, and noticed I was there, bubbly and smiling, at the start of the after-show parties, but at the end of the evening was always nowhere to be seen.

This was all part of a cultural landscape that was unthinkingly sexist and misogynistic. My first TV job was as a dancer on *The Benny Hill Show* in November 1984. The scripts were full of smutty, schoolboy humor and sexual innuendo. One of my onscreen cameos featured me in a so-called Victorian dress with a hole cut out at my cleavage, which Hill used as a stand for his menu card. That scene was broadcast on mainstream television.

Hill himself was a very sweet man who looked after the dancers who worked for him, but there were others around who pushed the boundaries of what they could get away with as far as they could. You might think this is all in the past, but as I have worked with younger women, I have been appalled to discover that even though on the surface society appears to have changed and women are given more rights and more agency, this kind of behavior has continued to be the norm. It might be more hidden, but for too long an actor or actress may well have been forced to behave in ways they didn't want to for the sake of their careers.

For decades, this dangerous dynamic has persisted, and

it reached a tipping point in 2017, when the allegations about Harvey Weinstein's persistent abuse and exploitation of actresses led to the launch of the #MeToo and #TimesUp campaigns. By this time, I was already in the thick of devising a code of practice that would improve the filming of scenes involving intimacy and nudity. I'd trained as an actor and had a family. From 2007, after earning an MA in Movement Studies at the Royal Central School of Speech and Drama in London, I worked as a movement director and movement teacher in five drama schools in London. As a result of my work on *Does My Sex Offend You?* in April 2015, I was invited by Meredith Dufton, head of movement at Mountview Academy of Theatre Arts, to develop a structure that would give guidance to actors when working with intimate content.

In researching the work, I was inspired and mentored by a colleague, Vanessa Ewan, who had already had the revelation that there should be a parallel between guidelines for staging a fight and those applying to intimate scenes. In her book *Actor Movement: Expression of the Physical Being,* co-authored with Debbie Green, she says: "There are methods to tackle these difficulties. Some are to do with the way the rehearsal or performance environment is managed, and in the absence of industry guidelines, they require commitment from the company or production team."[7]

The phrase "in the absence of industry guidelines" became my lightbulb moment. Why weren't there guidelines covering such an important aspect of our work? Why should actors rely on individual companies or producers to put the structures in place to provide a safe framework in which they could work? Why should that be the status quo? I thought, I can change that! I can share the ideas I am developing and help to create guidelines in an industry where they did not exist. Instead of making people take personal responsibility, why not try to make the industry change itself by adopting a code of best practice? I am very focused once I get an idea in my head, and I was seized with the importance of finding a way to give the film, television, and theater industry a new standard for how to create intimate scenes. That was in 2016.

So, in early 2017, I presented a version of the guidelines to various sectors of the industry and on July 12 of the same year to the Personal Managers Association (PMA) monthly meeting. On February 3, 2018, I was invited to present the Intimacy on Set Guidelines at the TIME'S UP UK women's committee, where they were instantly endorsed by Women in Film and TV (WFTV UK). Subsequently, they have been adopted across live performance, film, and television. On just over a single page, they share guidance for producers, directors, casting directors, agents, and actors. They cover the process from audition through rehearsal to performance. The overriding tenets of the Intimacy on Set Guidelines are: open communication and transparency, agreement and consent, clear choreography, and closure. You can read the entire document at the end of the book.

Without realizing it, I had created a new role for myself. As I shared the Intimacy on Set Guidelines and the thinking behind them, I was asked onto sets as an intimacy coordinator, working to improve conditions and develop new ways of staging intimate content. In 2018, the first three productions I worked on in that capacity were *Sex Education*, starting with a groundbreaking day's workshop on April 25, 2018; *Gentleman Jack*, which began on May 8; and HBO's *Watchmen* (the TV series), which started on September 13 of the same year. A new way of creating sex onscreen was up and running, and by the time *Normal People* aired in 2020, it was clear just what a difference it was making.

I have realized, as I have gone on my own journey in this new world, that some of what I have learned can be applied not only on the film set but in the real world too. A common misconception is that the work of an intimacy practitioner (which is known as intimacy pedagogy when teaching and intimacy direction in live performance or intimacy coordination in TV or film work) is confined to the bedroom scenes we see onscreen or onstage. But as with our own intimate lives, we know that it is the work we do beforehand, both with ourselves and with our partners, that creates the foundations for satisfying connection and truly intimate encounters. I want to focus on how some of the tools an intimacy practitioner uses to build trust and empower open communication can help us build stronger relationships everywhere in our lives.

As I've said earlier in the chapter, there are four overriding tenets of the Intimacy on Set Guidelines for the filming of intimate scenes. First is open communication, so that everybody knows what they are doing at any given point. Second, agreement and consent, which put in place firmly established boundaries, including agreed strategies to halt the action where necessary. Third, clear choreography for all intimate scenes. Finally, closure.

These are not bad starting points for the basis of a healthy relationship.

I joked earlier that I can't come into your bedroom and

choreograph your sex life, but we can all choreograph our lives to some extent. At its most basic level, choreography is the control of time and space to create pattern and meaning, and by using the techniques I've developed to build safety, trust, and openness on set, I can help you create a space where you feel connected to your body, so that you can experience your desires, communicate your boundaries, and hold space for your partner(s) to feel safe opening up with you. This kind of choreography, when applied to intimacy, can help to create powerful relationships, and also help us to understand more broadly the place we are at in our lives. You have the autonomy to create the design and purpose of your life to allow you to live as the best version of yourself. You give yourself the framework to connect with your body, to communicate your boundaries that allow your partners to feel safe communicating with you too. In this way, we can all create more powerful intimate relationships in our lives.

WHAT DO I WANT?

To begin the journey of creating more powerful intimate relationships, the first step is to set our intentions and ask ourselves really simple questions: *What do I want? What do I want in my intimate life? What do I want in my sexual relationships? What are my fantasies? What are my desires?*

In order to answer these questions meaningfully, it is helpful to take time out of our busy lives to pause, be quiet, and be present with ourselves. You can use techniques such as meditation, writing a stream of consciousness, or going for a walk to listen, think, and consider the answers that reveal themselves to you. This time-out gives you the space to be conscious of your starting place, and from there you can then take your first step toward what you want.

Every day, I work with actors and students to give them methods to discover the joy of being in the body, of feeling the sheer pleasure of breathing and being alive. I invite actors to put their mind in their breath and their breath in their body—to work with presence and mindfulness and engage their physical being.

One of the simplest and most effective tools that you

can use is the power of the breath, to take you from one state ready for the next, to allow you to pause and notice. The exercise I often use is called "20 connected breaths."

I've outlined the exercise on the following pages, and I'd like to invite you to read through it and then, as we begin this journey together, to experience the exercise yourself.

20 CONNECTED BREATHS

In my late twenties, I started working with a rebirthing practitioner. As a way of getting you ready, moving from your everyday self into the session, the practitioner would use a technique of 20 connected breaths. Twenty connected breaths are all you need to change your state of being from your everyday self to a place of centeredness and calmness, ready for the work at hand.

I have since used this exercise throughout my career, for example when teaching in drama schools if I had students coming in from a lunch break, incredibly excited for some reason. Instead of asking them to be quiet or settle down, all you need to do is invite them to sit on the floor, hands on their knees, and engage them with 20 connected breaths. At the end of which you have beautiful, calm students, ready to focus on the next part of the day.

This exercise is an important foundation in all of my movement work. I hope it will connect you with your body and breath and bring you to a place of calm and stillness.

Connected breathing means that each breath is connected to the last one, and also to the next one. There are no pauses or gaps between the breaths. The inhale turns into the exhale, and the exhale merges with the inhale. It is like a wheel turning. Inhale and exhale, exhale and inhale, each connected in a seamless circle to the other.

- Start by sitting comfortably, either on a chair or on the floor, with your back upright, head floating, or if you prefer, lying down. If you are sitting on a chair, sit toward the front of it so that you can have your feet placed firmly on the floor. If needed, put a cushion or blanket under your feet so you can be in the most comfortable position to sit with a straight spine.

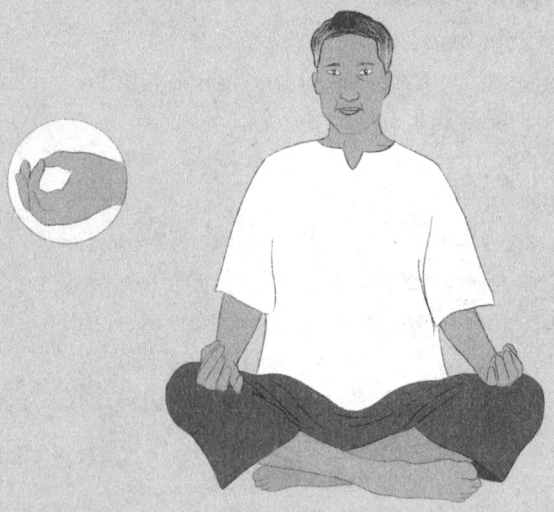

- Either hold a soft focus with your gaze, looking at a fixed point in front of you, or close your eyes.

- I shall talk you through the first 10 breaths, and then leave you to continue the next 10 breaths following your own focus.

- Throughout this exercise, breathe in through your nose, and breathe out gently through the mouth. While doing this, try to notice what is activated by the breathing. Let yourself be conscious of what you are doing. Keep your focus on the breath, and if you notice that the mind has wandered, that is fine. Just bring the focus back again to the flow of your breathing.

1. Start by taking a breath in through your nose, bringing your breath down deep into your belly, allowing your belly to expand.

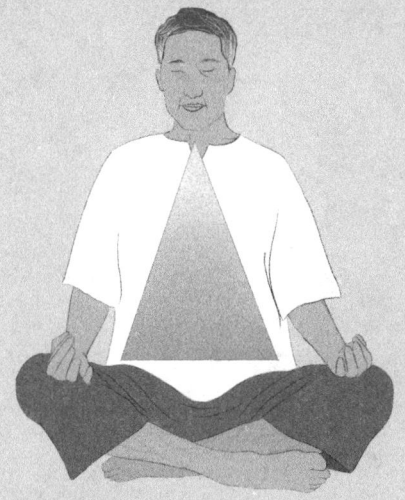

As you exhale through your mouth, feel that your head is floating upward on the out breath, lengthening your spine.

2. On the next inhale, breathe into your ribs, letting them expand in width. Enjoy the feeling of your breath filling the lungs.

On the exhale, once again feel your head floating upward, lengthening your neck and spine.

3. On the next inhale, notice your breath moving into your skull, feeling as though your skull expands in width.

   As you exhale, once again feel your spacious skull floating upward.

4. Inhale deeply again, breathing into your belly, allowing your belly to expand, and on the out breath, imagine that a root is growing from the tip of your coccyx, down into the earth.

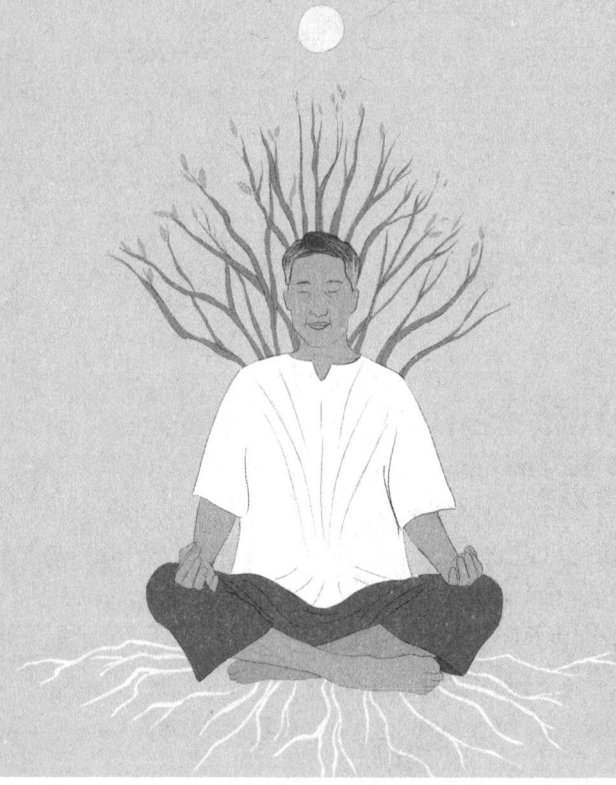

5. Repeat, inhaling deeply again into the belly, and on the out breath, imagine that the root is growing from the tip of your coccyx, farther down into the earth, wrapping around roots and boulders beneath you, anchoring you into it.

6. On the next inhalation, imagine that you're breathing all that earth energy in through that root, up through your coccyx and then your spine, allowing that energy to travel all the way up to the top of your skull.

   As you exhale, imagine now that there is a pinpoint in the top of your skull, and that when you breathe out, it shoots out of your head, going all the way up to the sun.

7. On your next inhalation, really breathe in that earth energy up through the spine, giving you weight and solidity. Enjoy the opposing sensations of your sitting bones and coccyx anchoring into the earth and your spine and skull pulling upward.

   On the next out breath, really imagine the breath flowing out through the top of the head up to the sun.

8. Now on the next inhalation, imagine you are bringing that fiery energy from the sun right into the top of your head, moving down through the spine to the coccyx.

   On the exhalation, send that fire energy from the sun down from your coccyx, down the root to the molten core of the earth.

9. On the next inhalation, breathe that earth energy up through the spine, and imagine sending it out through the top of the head as you exhale.

10. Inhale and bring the sun's energy down into your body once more, sending it down into the earth on the exhale.

- From there, continue with another 10 connected breaths in your own time. As you do so, imagine the breath moving through whichever parts of the body that feel good to you, and enjoy these beautiful sensations.

- When you have completed another set of 10 breaths, 20 in all, bring yourself back into the space.

- If your eyes were closed, open your eyes, look around you, and orient yourself back in the room.

- Stretch out and follow whatever impulses your body is asking for. Maybe you want to stretch your arms up over your head, or do a side bend, or stretch your legs and touch your toes. Enjoy the sensation of giving your body exactly what it wants and needs!

- Finally, focus on the next thing that you're going to do in your day, feeling more spacious, centered, and connected with your body.

Breathing is the first step to setting your intention about every aspect of your intimate relationships. Now you have come to that still place, you can really listen to yourself and ask some of these questions:

- *Am I happy with my intimate relationships?*
- *What aspects are working?*
- *What aspects fulfill me?*
- *What aspects no longer quite work?*
- *What aspects do I want to shift and change?*
- *Are my partner and I stuck in habits of decades? (If you have been lucky enough to be together for that long.)*
- *Are there things I could change that would deepen our intimacy?*
- *What kind of person do I want to meet? (If you are single.)*
- *What do I want from a relationship?*

A field guide is most useful if you know what you want.

Keeping this sense of presence and mindfulness has never been more important for all of us because as the twenty-first century progresses, we are becoming increasingly separated from the world around us. So many aspects of modern behavior separate us from each other. Sometimes when I am working with students, I suggest they take a journey on a bus, subway, or train and consciously watch the people around them. What you notice, if you are looking, is how little contact there is. People carve out a space for themselves with luggage and bags. They might sit with their legs apart, assertively marking their territory. They might shrink into the smallest area they can, keeping their elbows and legs within the confines marked out by the arms of their chairs.

Most people will be on their mobile phones, looking at the screen. Screens are arguably the greatest barrier to intimacy in the world today. We all focus on our phones, looking down, away from everyone else. In some ways, this is a means of self-preservation. We might not want to make eye contact with anyone else for all kinds of reasons. But it also makes it more difficult—in real life at least—to strike up any form of intimacy with another person. As I will explain in the next chapter, the first step to intimacy is often the gaze—that's hard to establish when you're looking at your phone.

Our increasing reliance on video calls and other forms of digital communication has also added a layer of complication. When you're talking face to face in the same room, you have a sense of each other's essence. You communicate viscerally in a way that you simply don't through a screen. I've had a few experiences when I have been talking through something with someone on a video call, then when we actually meet, I realize there is more depth to be gained from meeting in person. On a screen, it is more challenging to pick up the signals and clues of agreement or dissent in the same way you can when physically present with another person. You think you have connected, you think your eyes have met, but they haven't.

Dating apps don't allow for spontaneous in-person connection. Yet interestingly, amid the algorithms, a sense of informality manages to come into play. Justin McLeod, CEO of Hinge, a dating app that aims to get beyond the hook-ups of Tinder and into meaningful relationships, gave an interview to *The Times* in September 2022 in which he noted that Hinge users pictured in gyms don't do as well (only 3 percent of successful daters display gym photographs) as users with videos that establish more meaningful connections.[1] Women who smile but don't look directly at the camera in their photos are chosen, while men who do look straight at the camera but don't smile are also popular. This fits into the theory of the gender stereotype whereby women present themselves for approval while a direct stare from men suggests that they are looking at you and taking control.

A potential date will often also supply photographs of themselves with their friends. By seeing them in real relationships with people, a new observer can see who they are, can see their animation and how they react. They look at people interacting with their friends and can imagine how they would engage with them. One of the other difficulties of viewing a world through a screen is that it separates you from the unexpected, from unintentional yet meaningful encounters that build a sense of intimacy. Photographs of interaction help widen the perspective.

I am aware it may feel challenging to enrich and develop our intimate lives amid all these pressures. But I'm always very conscious that there are a lot of good people in the world, and a lot of happy relationships. However, young women are struggling to be able to be themselves without conforming to the dictates of social media and to be able to take their space in the world and call their boundaries. Our young men are often struggling to find their place, learning how to be in their masculinity and to inhabit themselves as men but also to be aware, sensitive, and caring, both in themselves and in their relationships. They are bounced around by social media that offers them all kinds of advice about virility and power, and they often feel they cannot win. If they are too dominant, they are considered to be overbearing; and if they are too gentle, they are accused of being a wuss.

There are certain qualities that tend to define successful relationships—whether between family, friends, or lovers. The website Teen Dating Abuse Awareness and Prevention offers a useful guide to what a healthy relationship looks like, and their suggestions apply for every age. Their characteristics include:[2]

- *respect for privacy and space*
- *partners encouraging each other to spend time with friends without them and to participate in activities they enjoy*
- *feeling comfortable expressing your opinions and concerns*
- *feeling physically safe*
- *your partner doesn't force you to have sex or do things that make you feel uncomfortable*
- *you respect one another's wishes and feelings, and can compromise and negotiate when there are disagreements or conflicts*

In later chapters, I'm going to go into detail about the whole business of setting boundaries and giving consent, but here I wanted to outline some of the other qualities I can bring from my work to the creation and maintenance of better intimate ties.

In traditional Indigenous cultures, where people essentially live in communication with the rhythm of life and with the flow of nature, there is often a sense of movement from one state to another, solving problems by embracing the cycle of nature.

I find it useful to think of a voyage when I am contemplating problem-solving and exploring issues in my practical and emotional life. Or to think of it more simply, you can imagine designing a dream home and thinking about what you want to achieve in the space you are living in and how the design can enable you to live your life the way you want. You can ask questions of yourself: How do you use your space at the moment? How does it make you feel? What do you want it to be? How would you ideally want to feel?

That sense of constant questioning, of traveling from one state to another, shifting and adapting to meet your needs and the requirements of others underpins healthy relationships.

When I check in with an actor, some of the first questions I ask them are: How are you feeling right now? Do you have any worries or any concerns? The purpose of doing that is to introduce a sense of presence and mindfulness, giving them an invitation to listen to their bodies, so they can be really in tune with their requirements and what their boundaries are. This helps obtain clarity as to their starting place for that day, and from there to make clear choices on how to proceed.

All of this marks huge progress from the past when in the entertainment industry, as in life, there has been a tendency to ignore people's personal boundaries. Troubling, neglectful, and abusive behavior has been inherent and systemic, sustained by the age-old idea of "Doctor Theater"—the idea that the show must go on, whatever the cost. In that expectation, you are basically saying you don't look after yourself or your needs, because the job comes first. You have flu, but you must perform however ill you feel. You fall on stage, but you jump up and keep going even though you've twisted your knee.

It has often been the case that the acting profession does not always accommodate the realities of life offscreen or offstage. I was in the audience at an interview at the Royal Central School of Speech and Drama when the actress Fiona Shaw was discussing just this. I was struck when she said that when she was a young actress in her twenties, her brother was killed in a car crash, at the age of just 18, and as she was rehearsing for her debut at the Royal Shakespeare Company, she needed to seek permission to attend his funeral. She added that the vocation of acting could, unlike many other jobs, keep one from friends, and recalled having missed several weddings due to her work commitments.

Perhaps a sign that things are getting better as time goes on, when Mark Rylance's younger brother died in a cycling accident in 2022, while he was performing Jez Butterworth's play *Jerusalem* in the West End, he took three performances off to attend his funeral in California— even though he was so important to the production that the show had to be canceled in his absence. He wrote to audiences explaining his decision: "I hope you understand my need to grieve my beloved brother and thank you for your support at this time."[3]

That felt to me like the coming of wisdom, of an acceptance that actually the job isn't everything. Life goes on outside the theater and outside the film set; people's needs must be attended to and cared for. This seems to me a lesson from my intimacy work that can be applied beyond the confines of film and theater. We all need to pay attention to ourselves and to our inner needs. Our work in whatever sphere can sometimes be so all-consuming that we fail to make space for ourselves. We can support and nurture ourselves by putting in place clear boundaries between our professional or public selves and our private lives.

There are simple techniques we can use to delineate a move from one section of our life to another. One of the difficulties of the times we live in is that the boundaries between professional and personal are often so blurred by the fact that our working lives seep into our homes. The omnipresence of cellphones means you can be contacted by the office at any hour of the day or night. The great societal changes brought about by the Covid-19 pandemic accelerated the idea of home working, so that people ended up hosting remote business meetings in their bedrooms, sometimes secretly still wearing pajamas.

Lockdowns because of Covid-19 forced us back into our homes, often in close proximity to others. It asked us to show different modes of ourselves—the friend, the lover, the parent, the cook, the office worker—all at the same time and in the same place. No wonder so many relationships came under pressure. No wonder the National Domestic Abuse Helpline in the UK reported a 65 percent increase in calls between April and June 2020, compared with the first three months of that year.[4] Even those of us lucky to live in largish spaces and who get on well with our partners found ourselves juggling multiple roles. I know I was aware of how important it was to be conscious of who I was at any given moment—the teacher, the intimacy coordinator, the advocate—and to be able to delineate when I stopped working and was in the role of mother or lover in my home with my loved ones.

In normal life, we inhabit different spaces assigned to those activities: We travel to the office to work or walk to meet a friend for a coffee in a café. We experience the liminal state of travel that transitions us from one place to another, from one state to another. Yet even then the sense of protecting space, of bookending the moment between a work and a leisure activity, of separating our public and intimate lives, is constantly under threat.

Bringing a sense of closure, of ending one thing before you begin another is important. To take an extreme example, during lockdown in 2020, I found myself in my study attending an online funeral while the daily business of domestic life unfolded in the rest of my home. We were all in the same house, but I was in a different place from my family because I was emotionally engaged in the service onscreen, literally in two places at once.

Metaphorically, the same thing can happen if you pass too quickly from one state to another, bringing all the concerns of your busy day at the office to your home life. I see it all the time with actors; if we have been filming a scene that is intense, involving, or perhaps upsetting, and they immediately step back into their lives, they can carry their work with them. Yet, in order to bring the best of yourself to any activity, your mind, body, intention, and emotion all need to be fully engaged with the task at hand. You have to be absolutely present to be the best of yourself.

It is always an idea in life to find a way of marking closure, taking a deep breath and a moment of stillness before you move on. One technique that is wonderful for this is the 20 Connected Breaths that I have already shared with you (page 27). Another technique I have found very useful is to suggest to actors that at the end of a day's work, they run their wrists under a cold tap, with their palms up, letting the water run on the lower forearm and at the same time allowing the energy of the scene and its emotional journey to flow away, drawing a line at the end of the working day with a physical gesture that allows them to return to their personal selves. You can use the same method in your life. Just try walking into the bathroom at the end of your busy day at work and allowing cold water to run over your wrists, consciously letting go of the preoccupations and concerns of the day, imagining everything flowing away, leaving you clear and cleansed, and in a state where you are ready to focus on the next part of your day.

Another technique is to light a candle while you work and to blow it out while you have a break or when you've finished a particular task. Simple rituals to support the conscious move from one mode to another allow us to respond to the demands of life and our relationships.

Another suggestion is to imagine you are under a waterfall and let everything that no longer serves you wash away. You might like to try the waterfall visualization exercise I've suggested on page 59.

All of these techniques help us to be conscious of where we are and what we might want. In terms of our intimate lives, expanding this sense of presence and mindfulness might mean we discover that we are aware of wanting something different and desiring something more in some way. You might want to take your relationship into new territory and new experiences. It's the same as when you decide you might want to go on a lifetime's holiday to New Zealand. In that instance, you would explore the different places in New Zealand online, look at maps, talk to your friends about experiences, and organize your travel. You would build a plan of the adventure.

That sort of planning is a kind of choreography, a gathering of information that enables you to create possibilities for what you want to happen next. It's the same in terms of our intimate lives. When we think about the experiences we might like to have with our partners, we can seek out sources to give us new ideas for the type of experience we'd like to create, which we shall go on to explore later in the chapter.

In our journey of discovery, as we forge intimate relationships and perhaps explore new territories, it's always worth being mindful of the fact that sometimes people pretend they know more than they do—or they withhold something vital from a conversation. Part of my role when I am working is to listen not just to what people are saying but how they are saying it, what language they are using and what is happening in their body. I look at what tensions they are holding. Sometimes—and this is a lesson for life as well as for my work—it is through silence or avoidance that people tell you what they don't like.

For example, I once worked on a play where the male character was choreographed to stroke the side of the female character's breast. The female performer had agreed this was fine with her, but when I watched them rehearse, time and time again, the male actor avoided the action. He hadn't said he was uncomfortable, but when we talked it through, he admitted he was not at ease with this intimate touch. We choreographed a different movement with which both actors were happy.

Similarly, at a table reading for a film, I noticed that it said in the script that a character would swim naked, but the actor playing the character spent a lot of time discussing the way in which they felt that this particular character would wear a swimming costume. I realized this was another way of saying that they didn't want to perform in the nude; after talking it through with the director, we found a different way forward for the scene. This is a very specific example, but it is also an instance of the way in which the observation skills I bring to my work on film reflect back into our lives. Imagine the person talking isn't an actor but someone you're in a relationship with and are inviting to do something with you. It might be a dance, or it might be a date. People sometimes find it very hard to say what they want, where they want to be touched or what upsets them.

As human beings, we naturally respond to other people's body language and impulses without even thinking. What I'm suggesting is that becoming more aware of how we read those signals can be a valuable skill for everyone. However, that skill starts with being consciously aware of how we are in our own bodies. In the next few chapters, I'm going to suggest ways that we can recalibrate our sense of self to enrich and enliven all aspects of our intimate lives.

Another factor that has an influence and impact on our intimate lives is the widespread availability of pornography that is now only a phone click away. People can be led to it from X (formerly Twitter) or TikTok, or just by typing the wrong suggestion into a search engine. You don't need to be searching for it to find it, but many people do seek it out and their increasing consumption of porn is having a distorting effect on their view of what is normal. In the absence of easily accessible, healthy education around sexual content, some people turn to pornography as the place to learn what sexual activity should be. In this way, the porn industry is inadvertently choreographing our sexual encounters, obscuring what we might want for ourselves.

The website Pornhub, one of the most popular online porn websites, has an estimated 50 million registered users and more than a billion sexually explicit videos uploaded for immediate viewing. In 2023, it reported more than 100 million visits per day and 2.14 billion visits during a single month, which is more than the combined visits to Netflix, TikTok, Pinterest, and Instagram. It is the fourth-most-visited site in the US, beaten only by Google, Facebook, and YouTube. The vast majority of viewers are men, but women are also looking to porn. Trends in porn also then gradually filter out into other forms of media and advertising, becoming a part of the cultural zeitgeist.[5]

If people watch pornography regularly, they are in danger of thinking that their sexual performance has to mimic what they are seeing, and that they must "perform" sexual intimacy at these unrealistic levels. They can be left feeling inadequate and unhappy. They can also become addicted, with repercussions in their sexual lives.

Conversely, it's also worth noting that at the same time that the internet is flooded by virtual sex, in our real lives, Covid-19 and fear of relationships have had a distancing effect. There is a long-term trend for people in general to have less sex with fewer partners. Dr. Justin Lehmiller, a Kinsey Institute research fellow and host of the *Sex and Psychology* podcast, puts this down to a variety of factors, including the use of dating apps as a means of finding partners. Online dating, he says, is an arena where "there's a lot of toxic behavior, brutal rejection and feelings of intense competition for mates. It can make sex and relationships feel like a high-stress, high-stakes thing."[6]

As a result, there is a well-documented rise in voluntary or intentional celibacy, which has become its own hashtag on TikTok. According to the article in the *Guardian* that quoted Lehmiller, by January 2023 #celibacy had more than 195 million views, with those who practice it claiming it has improved their focus, mental health, and energy. Among the reasons people give for avoiding sex is the pressure to hook up on online dates, the fear of rough sex encouraged by pornography, and a decline in alcohol consumption.

The combination of these factors means that young people are having less sex than previous generations. According to the same article, the National Survey of Sexual Health and Behavior in the US found that between 2009 and 2018, there was a rise in adolescents reporting no sexual activity (partnered and alone) from 28.8 to 44.2 percent of young men and from 49.5 to 74 percent of young women.[7] There's an odd contradiction here: rape culture is on the rise, thanks to pornography, but so is the sense that our young people either feel inadequate or so fearful that they won't even venture to have sex or attempt intimacy.

The Netflix comedy drama *Sex Education* provided a valuable picture of the pressures young people face as they discover their sexuality and feel their way into the complexities of relationships, without really having much clue what they are doing.

I was really proud to work on the first two seasons which, for the first time that I can think of, showed intimate encounters between young people in ways that were naturalistic, truthful, and often very funny. Otis (Asa Butterfield) is the son of a sex therapist played by Gillian Anderson, and with the encouragement of his classmate Maeve (Emma Mackey), he begins to offer sexual advice to his classmates, even though he himself is a virgin and deeply confused about his feelings for the girls in his life and his relationship with his own sexual anatomy and expression.

One scene in particular showed the effects of pornography when Aimee (played by Aimee Lou Wood) is trying to behave in ways that she felt she should behave when she was being sexual with her boyfriend "Top Heavy" Steve (Chris Jenks), writhing and breathing heavily, asking him if he wants to ejaculate on her face or her breasts. He stops her. "Do you actually want me to do any of that stuff?" he asks. She pauses and replies, "Yeah, I think so." But Steve goes on, "It feels like you are performing. Tell me what you want."

The encounter reveals the dangers of acting out the choreography that someone else has set for us, not discovering what we truly want. Aimee is encouraged to explore her own pleasure by wannabe sex therapist Otis, who acknowledges that women often feel more shame about masturbation than men. By discovering what really excites her and gives her pleasure, she is able to enhance her relationship and her own self-worth. She can come back and tell Steve exactly what she wants. "When I start to shake, blow on my ear and get ready for fireworks," she says. Steve looks happy but stunned. "I am on it," he replies.

I was really proud to help shape the masturbation montage scene. Anyone who watched it—both young and old—would have had a clear and humorous insight into the way that taking charge of the choreography of your own intimate life can led to a successful sexual encounter. I even had a student come up to me to say that that scene had "changed her life," that it had given her permission to have autonomy over her own body and allowed her to explore herself in ways that were prohibited to her before. It was so wonderful to receive such positive feedback.

I am not an expert in sexual content per se; I research each project to create an intimate vocabulary that's suitable for the film or play that I am working on. For example, when I was involved with the first season of *Gentleman Jack,* I looked at sofeminine's "Lesbian Kama Sutra: 100 Sex Positions for Women," which showed different potential sexual positions.

I would suggest that couples in real life could do worse than doing a bit of research themselves if they want to connect differently in their intimate life. The *Kama Sutra* is a brilliant source of ideas for shapes and possibilities that take you outside what you know—and there are many different versions now available. One of my favorites is *The Little Book of Kama Sutra* by Sadie Cayman because it has the clarity of cartoon drawings with shapes. It's fun and it's accessible. I'd suggest you do what I do: Go and look at some shapes. Try things. Instead of feeling that sex must always work from the inside out, from the emotions to the physical act, experiment with working from the outside in.

As Cayman explains in her disclaimer: "Summersdale Publishers cannot be held responsible for any injuries or breakages that may occur when following the advice of this book. Always check on your partner's wellbeing when trying new positions, and please enjoy yourself carefully!" That's exactly what I'm advocating. See which positions inspire you and gently try them out, possibly fully clothed first. It's like a game. You're not asking "Do I feel this?" You are opening yourself out into the joy and fun of exploration. You're using a book like this as a map to discover a new choreography for a sexy, intimate encounter.

You need to set all of this within a safe context and communicate with your partner about what you want and how you are going to call a halt if you don't like it. But if you set the right boundaries in place (and I will come to how to do that in a later chapter), then consulting guides can help you to find deeper connection, freedom, and play in your intimate life and move its expression onto a different plane. Search out expertise by looking at books or posters or videos—or simply by talking to someone who knows more than you do.

Once you have listened to yourself, and explored what you might want, you are in a better position to begin to build rewarding intimate encounters, to take the first steps toward intimacy.

BODY PLEASURING

I first encountered this exercise when I was getting an MA in Movement Studies at the Royal Central School of Speech and Drama; it is drawn from Lorna Marshall's practice as written out in her book *The Body Speaks*. This exercise is about connecting with your body. Once you allow yourself to experience the joy of being in your body, you get better at reading your impulses and knowing what is right for you and what makes you feel good.

• Start by lying down on the floor in a clear, open space and closing your eyes.

• Breathe in. Then as you breathe out, release your body into the floor. Feel your belly expand as you breathe in and then release as you exhale.

• On your next breath in, breathe into your skull and then exhale, releasing all the tensions from your forehead around your eye sockets, and your jaw down into the floor.

• Next, breathe into your rib cage and, as you exhale, release your all the tensions from your chest and your shoulder blades down into the floor.

• Repeat by breathing into your pelvis, then your legs, then your arms, releasing the tension from each part of your body after each breath.

• Now that you have fully released all of the tension in your body and you are feeling connected to the ground, focus on your legs and your hips for a moment. Keeping everything from your waist up still, allow yourself to move your legs and hips freely, and do whatever they are asking you to do, whether that's a jiggle, a shake, or a stretch.

- If, as you move, there is an urge to make any kind of sound, allow yourself to make it, all the while allowing your legs to make any movements they want, just feeling the joy of moving and of exploring the sensations in your body.

- Do this for about one minute (or longer if you need to), and then return to stillness, lying on your back with your legs and hips on the ground once again.

- Take a moment to notice how your legs and hips feel. What are they saying? Do they feel different, now that they have made the movements they wanted to make?

- Now bring your attention to your arms and your torso and your upper body. This time, keeping your hips and legs still, allow yourself to move your upper body freely, experiencing the pleasure of moving.

- Allow your upper body to move freely. Explore the movement of your arms and your torso. Continue to breathe as you stretch, shake, jiggle, squeeze, and float your upper body in any way you wish, and if you feel an urge to make a sound, allow those sounds to come out freely. All you need to do is listen to what your body wants to do.

- Repeat this for one minute, remembering to breathe deeply throughout.

- When you have finished exploring the movements your upper body is asking for, return to stillness, bringing your upper body back down to the floor and lying flat on your back.

- Once again, take a moment to reflect on how your body feels, noticing what feels alive and what feels connected, noticing what feels different.

- Finally, I invite you to complete the exercise by going into full-body pleasuring, allowing your whole body to move freely, connecting the upper body and the lower body, allowing the legs, hips, arms, head, and core to move freely, listening to what your body is asking for. You might roll. You might spiral, you might turn. Enjoy the feeling of movement, and allow yourself to jiggle and stretch and make sounds with no judgment. Do this for one minute before returning to stillness.

- Once you have returned to stillness, lie on the ground for a few moments and reflect on the idea of what gave you pleasure. What movements was your body craving? Which ones felt good in the body?

- Lie still, enjoying the connection with yourself. Feel connected to your impulses and consider which parts of your body feel newly known or that you have experienced differently.

- Slowly open your eyes, allowing yourself to come back into the room, and take all the time you need before sitting up and returning to your day.

BODY SCAN

A body scan is a really lovely opportunity to pause, to listen to and connect with your body. In this moment, there's nothing to do, nothing to change, nothing to judge. Instead, this is an opportunity to simply notice your body and become attuned to what it is telling you. This exercise can be repeated several times to deepen your connection to your body.

- Start by noticing where you are, noticing where you are connected with your body, where you are connected with the ground.

- Begin by standing with your feet hip-width apart. You can either have your eyes closed or you can hold a soft gaze on a point in front of you.

- As you breathe in, imagine that there's a beautiful golden ring floating an arm's length above your head.

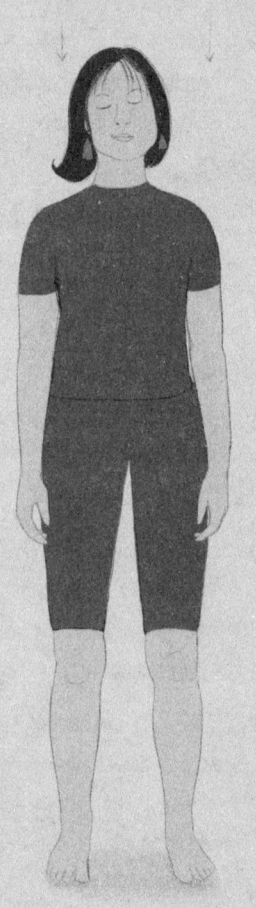

- As you exhale, imagine this beautiful gold ring is floating down toward your head. As it passes around your body, notice the different parts of your body.

- Continue to breathe in through your nose and out through your mouth as the ring slowly comes down.

- As the golden ring reaches the top of your skull, how does the top of your head feel? Are there any tensions there or in your forehead? How does the skin feel around your skull as the ring slowly cascades down?

- As the ring passes down, feel the tensions around your eyes and within your jaw, and feel how you are holding your lips.

- Continue to become aware of each part of your body as the golden ring continues downward. How is it feeling in the back of your neck and between your shoulder blades? What are the tensions in the front of your chest? How are you holding your stomach? How does it feel in the small of your back and into your buttocks? Which parts of your body feel tense, supported, or relaxed?

- Coming down to your legs, how are the tensions at the front of your thighs and your hamstrings? How are you holding your knee joints? How does it feel in your shins and the back of your calves? How does it feel down into your ankles and then into your feet? How much of your feet are in contact with the floor?

- And then allow the ring to come back up to circle each arm. How do your arms feel as they hang from your shoulders? What are the sensations in your upper arms, down into the line of your elbows, your forearms, and then your wrists? What is the curl of your fists?

- Gently touch your fingertips on your thighs, noticing where your hands hang and at what point they touch on your thighs.

- Where is your breath in the body? How deeply are you breathing? Where does the breath go?

- Now, notice where the heat is in your body. Where in your body is warm? Where in your body is cold?

- From there, I invite you to notice your impulses. As you notice your impulses, allow your body to follow your impulse wherever it may take you.

- Follow what feels good for your body—stretching, opening, jiggling, shaking. If there's sound that goes with those impulses, then invite that sound to be there. Allow yourself to make those sounds freely.

- As you stretch, give your body exactly what it wants, exactly what it desires.

- Next, allow your movements to become a little bit faster and a little bit more vigorous. I invite you to shake out any tensions in your body, starting by shaking your shoulders, letting any sounds you want to make come out freely.

- And then keep loosely shaking your body, down through your shoulders and your belly. Let your belly wobble freely for a few moments.

- Then lift up onto the balls of your feet and shake your whole body out, letting your face and your belly hang down.

- And then stretch your body right out into a beautiful X-shape, reaching your arms up and out widely, and feel a diagonal line running from your right foot through your belly button up to your left hand, and

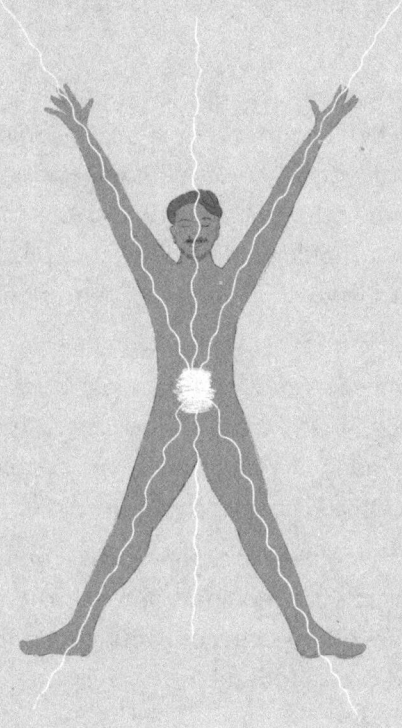

from your left foot through your belly button up to your right hand as you breathe in.

- As you breathe out, enjoy the full stretch of your body, extending your energy out into the space.

- Feel the space that's on either side of your body and the space in front of you and the space behind you.

- Next, drop your wrists, elbows, arms, and shoulders back to your sides, and release your head forward. Gently allow yourself to roll down, one vertebra at a time, feeling every vertebra on the way down, as the weight of your skull gradually pulls your spine down toward the floor, going as far as it's good for you to go.

- And as your head comes past your pelvis, allow your knees to bend so that your stomach comes onto your thighs with your head dropping down to the earth. Allow your upper body to drop down and then gently shake your shoulders. Feel like your arms are a big elephant's trunk snaking from side to side. Enjoy these lovely sensations.

- Once your arms and shoulders feel loose and relaxed, take a deep breath and, as you exhale, push your feet into the floor, rolling up slowly, one vertebra at a time, until your head is back on your shoulders.

- Roll your shoulders back three times. Bring your fingertips to your shoulders and roll your elbows back three times. Then throw out your arms and make three big, bold circles with them.

- Lower your arms, come back to center, close your eyes, and take a deep breath and have a moment of stillness.

- Now begin the second body scan. As you exhale, imagine the gold ring hovering at an arm's length above your head again and slowly coming back down.

- As it descends around your body, slowly pay attention to each part of your body and notice how you are feeling. What's the same, what's different?

- Notice the top of your skull, your forehead, your eye sockets. How is the back of your head feeling? How are you holding your lips and your jaw?

- What is the feeling at the back of your neck, and down into your shoulder blades?

- How does it feel at the front of your chest, and down into your belly? Are you holding it differently on this second body scan?

- Notice the sensation in your buttocks, and feel the front and back of your thighs as the ring keeps moving down around you.

- Next, we reach your knees. How are they feeling? Moving down into your shins and your calves, what's the same? What's different? How are you feeling in your ankles, and how are your feet in contact with the floor?

- Then, imagine the ring going down your arms from your shoulders to your fingertips. How do your shoulders feel? How are your upper arms and elbows?

Feel your forearms and your wrists. How do your hands feel?

- Once again, let your hands hang so that you feel the touch of your fingertips on your thighs. Are they hanging in the same place, or have they changed position in this second scan?

- Notice the breath in your body, and then notice the heat in your body; what feels warm and what feels cold now?

- Finally, close your eyes and stand still, and just notice how you feel in your body. Are there any parts of the body that you enjoyed moving, or any part of the body that you feel grateful for, or were even surprised about?

- Open your eyes. Bring yourself back into the space, grateful for the beautiful connection you've made to your body by acknowledging these sensations.

WATERFALL

This is an exercise for letting go. So often we pass from one moment to the next without stopping. I'd like to encourage you to pause as you transition from one part of your day to another, allowing your body and mind to process what might have passed and what might be yet to come. The waterfall is a great exercise to do this.

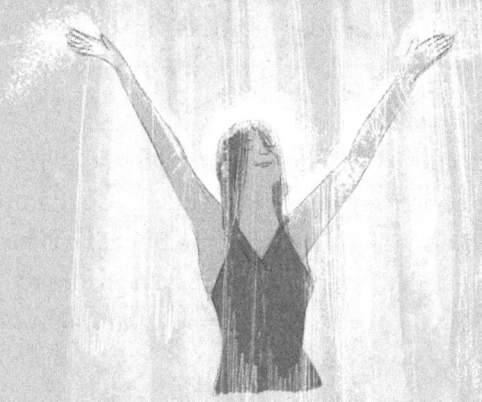

- As you come to closure at the end of your day, take a moment to acknowledge your feelings. What has resounded with you so far today, and what's been good for you? What aspects of the day, what moments do you want to take with you as you move forward? Imagine yourself holding those moments in your hands and bringing them into your heart for safekeeping. What aspects of the day do you want to let go of? Let's use this exercise to leave those things behind.

WHAT DO I WANT?

- Imagine you are standing under a beautiful crystal-clear waterfall with water cascading down over your head, and your feet are planted in a clear, cool pool with ripples around your feet.

- Now, you can begin to brush away what no longer serves you, allowing it to be carried away by the water.

- Bringing your hands up, you can use them to brush over your body. Moving your hands over your arms, over your belly, over your buttocks, imagine you are brushing that water off your body. Continue to breathe deeply.

- Moving to your lower body, now have a sense of water washing away down your thighs, down your hamstrings, down your calves, and imagine the beautiful clear water washing away now that you have cleansed yourself. As you do, allow the things you want to let go of to slip away with the water.

- As everything washes away, enjoy that wonderful sense of feeling cleansed, and having let go of everything that you don't want to take forward for the rest of the day.

- Gradually open your eyes and return to the moment.

- Take a step back, as though you are taking a final step back away from what you want to let go of.

- Now you're ready to take on the next part of your day.

CHAPTER THREE

THE FIRST STEPS TOWARD INTIMACY

I think it's important at this point to be clear about what intimacy is—and what it isn't. As I mentioned in the prologue, intimacy is not the same as sex, although in the right circumstances, it can lead to sex. There are different types of intimacy: physical, sexual, emotional, intellectual, spiritual, and experiential. You can be intimate with someone without ever touching them, though you might feel the need to touch as your intimacy grows.

Some of the closest relationships are in families, between parents and children and between siblings. In the same way, friends might have an intellectual intimacy, or a creative intimacy that has nothing to do with physical attraction and everything to do with the meeting of minds. The Greeks had multiple words for love, such as *eros, philia,* and *agape,* that described the varying qualities of love, which was a concept pondered over by some of history's most famous philosophers, including Plato and Aristotle.[1]

But it's probably true to say that in all cases—between

eventual lovers, between friends, between a mother and a child—the beginnings of intimacy lie in the gaze, that first flicker of eye contact that sparks a reaction. It's certainly true that when I am sent a script, I always look for the moment when the characters who will eventually become lovers first encounter one another. For example, when I worked on Laure de Clermont-Tonnerre's 2022 film adaptation of D. H. Lawrence's novel *Lady Chatterley's Lover*, the challenge was to imagine and choreograph the arc of passion between the aristocratic Lady Chatterley, played by Emma Corrin, and the gamekeeper Mellors, played by Jack O'Connell.

This was a relationship that was so transgressive when the book first appeared in 1928 that it was published in an unexpurgated form in England only in 1960, after a famous obscenity trial. Nowadays, people aren't so easily shocked by an explicitly described love affair across class barriers, but the relationship is still the heart of the story. Both characters find liberation because of it, so the challenge was to find ways of showing each beat of its development onscreen for the audience to understand its significance.

As a book and as a film, *Lady Chatterley's Lover* is about unlocking the intimate life. When we first meet Constance Chatterley, she is a young bride. She's bohemian, warm, open, and longing for physical contact. Her husband, Clifford, is uptight, frigid, and frightened. Once they are married, Clifford is injured in the trenches, paralyzed, and confined to a wheelchair; Constance ends up being his caregiver, further distancing her from the close intimate relationships she longs for. It's in this context in the screen version that she first sees Mellors as she watches him playing with his dog. He doesn't see her, but that is the moment intimacy is initiated—as she watches him. Later, he observes her washing her face in a stream. There's a spark of something on both sides. For me, the way they both furtively watch one another is the beginning of their story.

If you think about what you like, what you are into, what you find attractive, there is always a spark that ignites your interest, how you might like someone or even lust after them. You might be watching someone who you find physically attractive, or you might be drawn by the skill they have, or the way you see them interacting with other people that gives you an insight into who they are and makes you want to find out more.

People often say that the eyes are the window to the soul. If we gaze too long into someone's eyes, either it can be seen as an act of aggression—a confrontation—or it can allow us to make a deep connection with that person. As we stare into someone's eyes, if we are attracted to them our pupils dilate and we release oxytocin, the hormone associated with bonding and trust. This is a beautiful and powerful nonverbal communication. But even if we don't desire someone, that gaze can be a means of dropping through layers of possible prejudice, assumption, and fear to allow us to see the humanity in the other person.

I have always been struck by Amnesty International's Look Beyond Borders project, which brought recently arrived refugees from Somalia and Syria and their European hosts together in a warehouse in Germany and asked them to look into one another's eyes for four unbroken minutes. They came away from the encounter with a new sense of connection. The idea grew from an experiment conducted by the psychologist Dr. Arthur Aron, who also devised a series of questions that he believed would help people fall in love. The empathy and compassion people display for each other after such encounters is striking, breaking through the barriers that separate them.

One of the intimate encounters I often think of when I am imagining ways of helping build a sense of intimacy onscreen is one witnessed by some 20 million people on YouTube.[2] In 2010, the conceptual artist Marina Abramović created a performance at the Museum of Modern Art in New York called *The Artist Is Present.* In a red dress that covered all of her body except her face and hands, she sat at a wooden table for eight hours a day, silently meeting the gaze of strangers who came to sit opposite her.

It was the most extraordinary undertaking in itself, but on the opening night of its three-month run, her former lover Ulay was present in the audience. From their first meeting in 1976, they had been artistic and life partners for 12 years, creating groundbreaking and daring work together, including an installation where he held an arrow at her heart. Then, in the middle of a plan to walk across the Great Wall of China, they split up. From that point, they didn't see or speak to each other for 22 years until the night he turned up in New York and sat opposite her at the table, nervously stretching his legs and adjusting his jacket. What happened next broke the internet. It gets me every time I watch it and fills me with the beauty of their relationship with each other.

He preens slightly, getting ready to be in front of her. As she opens her eyes and sees him opposite her, they smile, and tears fill their eyes. It is utterly beautiful. As they reconnect with each other, you can see their emotions: Their bodies just fizz with delight, surprise, memory, love, hurt, pain. Everything is there. There's a purity in their emotion that we the audience—in the room, or from a computer/phone screen—are being allowed to witness. There's sexual tension, but there's also friendship, peace, and acknowledgment.

Then Abramović breaks her own rules. She leans across the table and lightly holds Ulay's hands. As she pulls her hands back, he leaves his hands there for a moment more, before pulling back and leaving. That's it. She closes her eyes and prepares for the next encounter. Of course, the moment had a follow-up—a whole other story that then unfolded between them. But what fascinates me is how perfectly that initial encounter illustrates the unspoken way that intimacy is communicated. Abramović has set up the space very carefully. She creates a performance area around herself that the audience cannot breach. In this she is explicitly exploring something that everyone does naturally. We all come with an inbuilt sense of our own kinesphere, a bubble of imaginary space that surrounds us. When people meet, they tend instinctively to keep themselves an arm's length apart. Abramović placed a table and chairs to mark the performance area; the chairs were placed approximately six feet apart, with the table in the space between.

One effect of Covid-19 was to make us all adopt this distancing behavior; if you are standing two arm's lengths away from someone—the six feet recommended by some scientists as a way of avoiding contagion—then you are immediately doing something that feels strange, that separates you from others. This means we circle one another rather than engaging. Covid made us fearful; it had the tendency of pushing us away from natural moments of closeness. We saw people separated from their elderly parents behind the glass of a nursing home window; we saw it in the streets and parks as groups of friends stood awkwardly apart from each other, trying to communicate, frightened to touch, anxious not to step into anyone's space. Those hesitations have left their residue today.

We've become less attuned to reading real spaces. Young people in particular, and perhaps all of us to an extent, can feel unmoored, less physically literate in being able to read micro gestures and more uncomfortable in our social encounters.

The truth is that if you are standing or sitting a single arm's length away from another person, you are both surrounded by imaginary protective spheres; you sense that the perimeters of your personal space are touching but as long as no one takes a step forward, your privacy and your boundaries are preserved (for more on these spheres, see the kinesphere exercise on page 132). As soon as someone moves forward into your space, something is beginning to happen. In the social dance that unfolds, if one person doesn't welcome the advances of the other, then they are likely to step backward to preserve their invisible bubble. But if they stand still, or move forward, then that sudden closeness alters the nature of the interaction, whether it be love or aggression, whether they are welcoming an encounter of a closer kind or standing up to it, ready to fight.

One of my earliest movement direction jobs on film was assisting the movement director Dan O'Neill on a sci-fi television series called *Humans,* which imagined a world where "synths"—highly sophisticated robot servants—had transformed society. In the development of the parameters in which the "synths" would operate, Dan realized that one way to show which actor was a robot and which was human was that robots wouldn't be able to pick up signals about personal space. They would stand facing someone, looking at them directly; that in itself is confronting. We don't stand absolutely square on to someone unless we actively want to be threatening. We tend to look or move away. We soften the lines of our bodies into diagonals, or sink slightly into our hips, showing that we are being friendly rather than aggressive.

To go back to *Lady Chatterley's Lover*, the first time Mellors and Constance touch in the film is accidental. They are handling chicks in Mellors's hut in the woods, both intent on caring for the birds. Interestingly, at the same time I was working on *Lady Chatterley's Lover*, I was involved with *Empire of Light*, the Sam Mendes film starring Olivia Colman and Micheal Ward, and that—quite coincidentally—has a similar moment of electricity, when their hands touch as they care for an injured bird. Both scripts reflect something that happens in life: As I have explained, in caring for something or someone else, you show something of yourself. The same logic applies to people who post online photographs of their interactions with their pets, which invariably attract multiple likes. Caring for an animal can show others the connection of your heart and in many ways gives a window into the essence of who you are.

It's important to recognize that what people consider intimate and appropriate is dependent on culture and religion. Attitudes to touch are conditioned by this. In the 1960s, the psychologist Sidney Jourard studied conversations in cafés between friends in different parts of the world. In England, the couples never touched. In the

US, they touched twice, once to say hello and once to say goodbye. In France, the number rose to ten touches in an hour, while in Puerto Rico, the friends touched each other 180 times. For Jourard, in our maddeningly crowded world, touch may be our salvation. "I think that body contact has the function of confirming one's bodily being," he says. "We live in an age of 'unembodiment' or disembodiment, and I believe that the experience of being touched enlivens our bodies and brings us back to them."[3]

Cultural differences are reinforced by religious practice. For my Muslim students, it is a huge barrier to climb when you ask them to hold hands; there is no way that they would kiss, even as part of training to be an actor. In life, and at work, I am always mindful of culture, religion, and religious constraints. We live in a world where we are becoming increasingly multicultural as movement across the globe increases, and societies become ever more mixed. This has resulted in many more multicultural couples and relationships. This joyous development means we have to get better at navigating different cultural preferences, honoring someone's culture or religion, and celebrating and incorporating everyone's differences. This obviously requires tolerance and flexibility all round.

But I am also conscious that, in general, we are getting far less physical in the way we live our lives—and the lack of physicality is accelerating. Twenty-odd years ago, I placed my own children on a mat under a baby arch and encouraged them to begin to explore the world by looking at the objects hanging over their head, concentrating on new shapes and different sensations. Now there are bouncer seats with iPad holders attached and baby toys that mimic a mobile phone. Parents give their toddlers phones to watch cartoons as a way of keeping them quiet. Before they can even walk, babies are being encouraged to experience the world through a screen! A study by the University of Iowa revealed that half of toddlers between 12 and 17 months could use an iPad by the age of one; 90 percent of the two-year-olds studied had mastered the gadget.[4]

When my children met other children as youngsters, they would still play outside, climb trees, and scuff a ball around. Increasingly, today's youngsters meet and play video games together; they don't even have to be in the same place. They can play alongside each other over the internet, separate yet together. The nervous energy courses through their bodies as they play; they imagine they are kicking a ball or leaping a wall, but in fact they are just sitting on a sofa, quite often alone, with their thumbs twitching as they guide their avatar with the device's controls.

Although precise data on the effect of screentime on child development is still being collated, one study of children between the ages of one and three from 2019 by the National Institutes of Health in the US discovered that children's average daily time spent watching television or using a computer or mobile device increases from 53 minutes at age 12 months to more than 150 minutes at three years.[5] Children who reported more than two hours a day of screentime got lower scores on thinking and language tests. Researchers also discovered that children with lots of screentime had a premature thinning of the outermost layer of their brains (the cerebral cortex), the area that supports the highest-order cognitive functions.

Terrifying though this is, screentime doesn't just alter

children's minds; it affects their bodies too. The result of an overreliance on entertainment provided through a screen, combined with other societal factors such as the loss of green open space, leads to a decline in physical activity, which accelerates as children grow up. This is a worldwide trend. Research published in the medical journal *The Lancet* in 2020 using data from 146 countries and 1.6 million students aged between 11 and 17 showed that 81 percent were insufficiently active. We are becoming separated from our physical bodies.[6]

This is combined with a growing disconnect about the actualities of life and death. My mum grew up on a farm and as a child, I used to go out to help my Uncle Pat milk the cows and we'd come back with a warm jug of milk that we'd use all day. When my granny wanted to cook chicken, she would go out to wring the chicken's neck and pluck it. The distance we often feel from our own physicality is the same distance between that lifestyle and walking to the corner shop for a pint of milk or to the supermarket for a prepacked chicken in a bag. In a similar way, when I was growing up—which is only a generation ago—there was a tradition in the Irish villages that my family came from that after someone had died, the family would hold a wake, where the body of the departed stayed in the house among the living. People were invited to come and pay their respects by the coffin, to touch the body and say their final farewells. I feel we shy away from that now. More people die in the hospital, and even if they die at home, death is professionalized, with undertakers whisking away a body as soon as breath has left it. When my father was dying, in the months when he was at home needing 24-hour care, I was conscious that we reestablished a relationship of touch that

I hadn't had with him ever, even in childhood. During his final illness, I was able to massage his swollen feet and legs to give him some relief, expressing my love for him by soaking his feet and cutting his toenails.

Families touching each other as they care for each other is another kind of intimacy. Simply doing things together—going out to eat, going swimming, going for a walk, even watching TV—tightens our bonds of connection. In relationships, shared activities and sensations are an important part of building true, deep intimacy that includes sexual and emotional intimacy but also reaches beyond that. I have always liked this quote from Antoine de Saint-Exupéry: "Love does not consist of gazing at each other, but in looking outward together in the same direction." Staring deep into each other's eyes might take you so far, but it also might lead to a codependent relationship where the outside world has lost its meaning. The kind of togetherness where you easily share the same experience, the same view, is just as important. That's why every night when my partner and I are in the same place, we try to walk outside and engage in a nighttime stretching routine, reaching up to the stars. It's a ritual that marks our connection with the ground, with the sky, and with each other. It's a kind of spiritual intimacy.

The common thread that unites all these thoughts is a sense of embodiment. It's something that can easily be lost in our busy lives—and it is also something we can seek to restore. By using some of the techniques I employ with actors, I invite you to cultivate an awareness of being in your own body, which can support you in nurturing your intimate relationships.

Embodiment can begin with doing very simple things

just to revive your sense of self in the world. Every day, for example, I try to walk barefoot on the grass, letting my skin make contact with the surface of the earth. It is a literal way of grounding myself, of absorbing the earth's natural healing energy.

Studies show that walking barefoot in this way has a variety of beneficial effects. One 2012 study points out that throughout history humans mostly walked barefoot or with footwear made of animal skins.[7] Through direct contact with the earth, the ground's free electrons were able to enter the body. "Through this mechanism, every part of the body could equilibrate with the electrical potential of the earth, thereby stabilizing the electrical environment of all organs, tissues and cells." Arguments in favor of it include better sleep, reduced muscle pain, and an improvement in general well-being.

There's no doubt that it makes you feel better, allowing you to feel the energy running up from your feet and into the body. As you get more stressed, your body is polarized like a magnet, charged into positive and negative ions. Walking barefoot on the grass releases the stress that has built up by literally grounding you, balancing out your energy. We'll talk more about being grounded toward the end of this chapter.

When I'm working with actors, we generally start with an exercise of this sort, just standing, feeling our feet on the ground, moving the weight of our bodies around so that it activates each part of the foot. Sometimes, I might suggest that they massage their own feet (see page 88). Then we will take time to connect with our breath using the exercise I described in Chapter Two.

It always sounds a bit odd to say that you need to

connect with your breath, because obviously the act of being alive means that we are walking around breathing every day. But what I am trying to do is to cultivate an awareness. As I've said, you put your mind in your breath and your breath in your body. Most of the time, unless you do a manual job, you're sitting down, using words to communicate, living in your head. Onscreen meetings, computers, phones, all of them mean that we might as well be heads on a stick, that our bodies aren't engaged in any way. If we stand up, roll our shoulders, shake our hands and our legs, then we are actually bringing our intention into our bodies. We are deliberately waking up the nervous system.

Since ancient times people have understood that there are different energy centers in the body. From their origins in Hinduism, these are called chakras, and they are widely used across various spiritual and holistic practices. The stresses and strains of life pull us off balance in various ways, either having too much energy or emotion or too little. Understanding our energy centers and employing movement, sounding, or meditation techniques to tune into those energy centers and bring balance helps us to live a healthier life.

The concept of the chakras is that there is a physical body and an energetic body. You'll find definitions vary, but broadly they identify seven centers in the body with their relevant emotions and attributes. This links with the examination of the endocrine system in Bonnie Bainbridge Cohen's Body-Mind Centering (BMC), which I studied and have been much influenced by.[8] Taken together, for me, they offer a way of understanding the relationship between our emotions and our physicality. You can work in life with the chakras on any level you like. You can feel the energy running up and down the spine or you can simply be aware of the journey from your dense body, rooted in our sensuality and sexuality, to the spiritual. You can see how someone feels about themselves in terms of how they hold their body, their posture and whether they are collapsed in that area or pushing forward in a particular place, or in a place of balance.

You can see the position of the seven chakras in the diagram on page 76. The base or root chakra, in line with the coccyx, is linked with "the instinct for physical creativity, unity, and the expression of shared sensuality, sexuality, and physical love"[9] as well as our primitive energy and a sense of survival. For men, this point represents the sexual energy of the gonads. For women, it is their base sexuality. In terms of the endocrine system, it is the adrenal glands that are associated with the life force, the instinct for survival, and the coccygeal body (a small, irregularly shaped cluster of cells lying at the tip of the tail bone), which "connects us to our roots within the earth, giving a groundedness that is based on self-love and the will toward personal survival, and that underlies instinctual love."[10] Its color is red.

The next chakra, located three finger widths below the belly button, in line with the sacrum, is the sacral chakra, the source of emotional energy, the belly brain that is the emotional connection within us. Significantly, since a women's sexual organs are the womb and the ovaries, which is the endocrine gland for this chakra, it also aligns with their sexual organs rather than being right down in the base area. That is why women's sexual energy is so often emotional. This energy center is about creativity and pleasure and is usually represented with the color orange.

Lifting to the solar plexus chakra, just below the diaphragm, is the sense of self, self-esteem, and self-confidence. We can either be in balance, or have low self-esteem and collapse in this place, or have an over-inflated sense of self where we extend out, pushing into space. The energy of the pancreas is the gland of the solar plexus chakra, which can "express strong emotional energies, such as anger, fear, excitement, and exuberance."[11] Its color is yellow.

Next is the heart chakra, the place of compassion, kindness, and our love: how we love ourselves, how we love others, how we allow ourselves to be loved. Its color is green. Lifting to the throat chakra, which is blue, it is our quality of expression, communication, and truth—how we speak out and are heard in the world. In terms of the endocrine system, it is the thyroid gland which "supports the power of the voice in singing" and is "the center of artistic and creative expression."[12] Then there is the third eye chakra in the center of the forehead, which aligns with the pituitary gland. Its color is indigo, and it is the place of our intellect, intuition, imagination, and perception. The final chakra is the crown chakra, which establishes the connection with our spirituality. It is represented with the color violet and links in the endocrine system to the pineal gland.

When physically warming up the body, I often focus on connecting with the spine as the most simple and clear image to connect with the energy centers through the body.

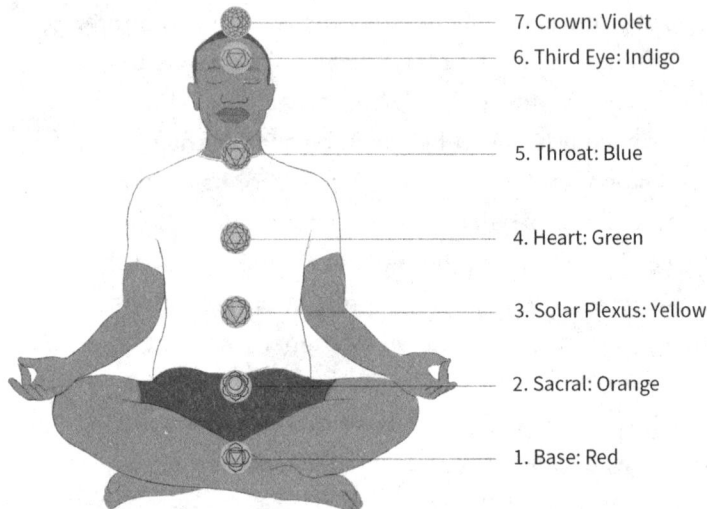

7. Crown: Violet
6. Third Eye: Indigo

5. Throat: Blue

4. Heart: Green

3. Solar Plexus: Yellow

2. Sacral: Orange

1. Base: Red

1. Coccyx (base chakra, red)
2. Sacrum (sacral chakra, orange)
3. Lumbar spine (solar plexus chakra, yellow)
4. Thoracic spine (heart chakra, green)
5. Cervical spine (throat chakra, blue)
6. Skull (third eye chakra, indigo)
7. Top of the head (crown chakra, violet)

If you imagine following the chakras up your body through these energy centers, the different connections are self-awareness, self-respect, self-worth, self-love, self-expression, self-responsibility, self-consciousness. When I am working with actors, we wake up the body through these energy centers, articulating through the spine, first as themselves, and then as their characters. What actors learn to do is to embody these emotional and energetic centers in their performance. If a character is timid and has low self-esteem, we would explore how they perhaps pull back in an area of the collapsed solar plexus. Or if they are playing a university professor who is focused on their work with ideas, reading, and intellect, we might work on placing the energy up in their head with that inner-seeing and a disconnect with the rest of their physicality. When I am choreographing intimacy, we always work from deciding the character's intention and main obstacle: what they desire in a relationship, what is stopping them from getting what they want, and where both of those sit in the body.

I often use a very brief moment of the first kiss in the scene from *Normal People* that we have discussed to explore an initial moment of intimacy. So many different types of intimacy are on display here. The first is intellectual, as Marianne is probing and questioning how Connell feels, wanting to understand his thinking and how he might be feeling about her. Connell is struggling to connect with his feelings and is interested in and amused by the banter with Marianne as they flirt with each other. As Marianne questions further, she is opening herself up with the question, "And what about now?" possibly dropping to the heart space, or to feelings of lust and desire.

MARIANNE
"So how do you know what you want?"

CONNELL
He pauses before replying.
"I don't. Most of the time I don't have a clue."

> MARIANNE
> *She turns her head and looks at his profile. She's thoughtful and serious.*
> "And what about now?"

> CONNELL
> *He moves toward her. They share a long look. He kisses her. They put their arms around each other, press their bodies against one another.*

> MARIANNE
> "Can we take our clothes off now?"

> CONNELL
> *He smiles. Tiny, amused shake of the head.*
> "Yeah."

An actor can choose different ways of playing that moment—but whatever they decide, it will show in their posture, in their body language. Perhaps Marianne loves Connell, so her actions are led by her heart center. Perhaps she physically desires him, so would energetically drop down into her sexual energy in the sacral chakra. However, she might be afraid of rejection and so be pulling back in the solar plexus center where she lacks belief in herself, waiting for the response from Connell to let her know the next step. For Connell, perhaps he finds the intellectual conversation allows him to connect with a side of himself that he cannot express at school, and this is what excites him, energetically connecting to the head center, and then once he follows this impulse, his sexual desire is ignited and and he too drops to the Sacral Chakra. There are so many choices that could be played here as the young teenagers explore the beginning of an intimate sexual relationship.

In terms of dramatic technique, actors train themselves to think and feel in different areas of the body so that the energy moves through the body depending on their choices. They activate the nervous system and the energetic journey, so you can see the impulse when you watch. In life, if we give ourselves the time and space to drop into our bodies and be more aware of what we are feeling, it brings our focus and attention to where we are at any particular moment of the day.

If throughout the day you try to maintain an awareness of how you are feeling and where those feelings are sitting in the body, you begin to understand yourself at a far deeper level. The first time I learned the Alexander Technique in the 1980s, my teacher, Ilan Reichel, told me to lie on the floor and actively listen to what my body was telling me, how I was feeling in my breath, focusing on where the tensions were, concentrating on each energy center. He called it "active listening."

Actively listening to our body in this way and recognizing the different energy centers helps us to understand what we are feeling, and by observing others, what other people are feeling about us.

In every kind of intimacy—spiritual, sexual, intellectual, or familial—recognizing in ourselves and others those subtle shifts, waking our bodies up so we have a sense of ourselves, gives us a better chance of being in sync with people we meet and being able to communicate more effectively in our personal and intimate life.

If you extend that process out into the world, into your interactions with people in your office, or at a social event or in a shop or with your loved ones, it helps you to be in an authentic relationship with the people you encounter. Active listening is being aware not just of what someone says but how they say it, the language that they are using, the tensions that are in their body as they are saying it, and how you are feeling as you are engaging with them. All of that helps us to be present and is an invaluable tool for meaningful relationships. We get as much, or more, information from nonverbal communication as from what someone actually says.

All of this is about connecting with our inner emotional landscape, our impulses, and our instincts about other people. However, a big part of how we present ourselves to the world is not about how we feel but how we look, the image we believe we have to present to conform to what is expected of us. That's the subject of the next chapter.

EYE GAZING

This exercise is an opportunity to connect with your partner, to explore and be really present with them. The exercise consists of three rounds of telling each other what you observe, what you notice, and then what you wonder about each other. There is nothing to judge, nothing to change. It's about sharing and receiving and experiencing this moment together. Before you begin, take a moment to agree on shared boundaries for engaging in this exercise; for example, that might mean avoiding sexual observations and not referring to any body parts in a sexual manner.

When you observe, share factual details about what you see. When you are being observed, remain silent, listen, and reflect on any sensations that arise.

- In the first round, observe and spend 60 seconds sharing your observations aloud.

- Then your partner will take their turn to observe you for the same length of time.

- Before moving on to the second round, take a moment of stillness, bringing awareness to any thoughts, feelings, or sensations that may have come up.

- In the second round, as you notice aloud for another 60 seconds, you can start to bring in more subjective elements, describing how your observations are painting a picture of your partner in this present moment. Has anything changed since the first round of this exercise?

- Then your partner will take their turn to notice you for the same length of time. As you are being noticed, sit in the moment, experiencing any thoughts or feelings that come up for you.

- Before moving on to the final round, take a moment to sit silently together and notice any thoughts, feelings, or sensations that may have arisen.

- In the final phase, you can reach out with your imagination and share what you are wondering about your partner. Once again, take 60 seconds, and begin, "I wonder . . ." before sharing your wonderings.

- Then your partner will take their turn to wonder about you for the same length of time. When you are being wondered about, let the thoughts hang in the air and experience how it feels to sit in the moment of wondering.

- When you have finished, take a moment in silence to reflect on your experience of the exercise.

- Sit with your partner and first talk about the experience itself before allowing the conversation to open up between you.

- When you have finished, you may choose to complete the experience together with a closure such as a hug.

WALKING BAREFOOT

Our feet are so important, both in carrying our weight and in connecting us to the earth. In this exercise, I hope to draw your attention to your feet so we can appreciate everything they do for us and feel better connected to them and therefore the earth.

I'd like to offer you a chance to walk barefoot. Walking barefoot outside in nature, on the grass, brings an amazing sense of connection, grounding you, connecting your neural pathways with the earth, allowing you to absorb the earth's natural energies. This can help to dissipate the tensions in the body, bringing a sense of calm, reducing stress and anxiety, and promoting a sense of well-being.[13] It's a really wonderful exercise. However, if you can't go outside, it's still beautiful just to connect with your feet and to walk barefoot wherever you are.

We all get stressed in our lives, and when we do, the energy in the body charges up like a magnet. How it works is that the earth's surface is rich in free electrons. When you walk barefoot, these electrons transfer to your body, neutralizing the positively charged free radicals. A really good way to de-stress yourself is to go out and connect with nature so that you can dissipate those positive and negative ions, like a lightning bolt finding its way to earth. One way of doing this might be to hug a tree that acts like the conductor, allowing your energy to go down into the ground. Another way of doing this is to walk barefoot on grass, sand, over rocks, or the earth.

Gaining an understand of the anatomy of the feet really helps you appreciate everything that they do for you. As you stand, your weight is centered on three points of your feet: the head of metatarsal 1, i.e., your big toe joint; the head of metatarsal 5, i.e., your little toe joint; and the center of your calcaneus, i.e., your heel bone. Please see the diagram of the foot and the points described below.

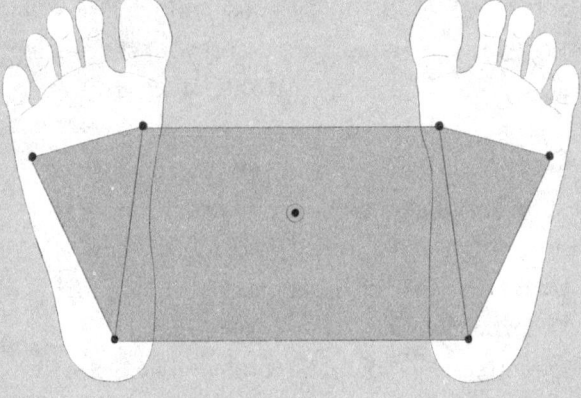

The arches of the foot are constructed like the arches of a cathedral, acting as a natural shock absorber, distributing the impact of your movements. The medial and lateral longitudinal arches run from the center of your calcaneus to the head of metatarsal 1 and the head of metatarsal 5, respectively. Your transverse arch is the curved arch across the middle of your foot, which goes right across the foot and has the height at the instep.

Finally, it is useful to think of the foot in two parts: the ankle foot, which is involved in weight bearing and

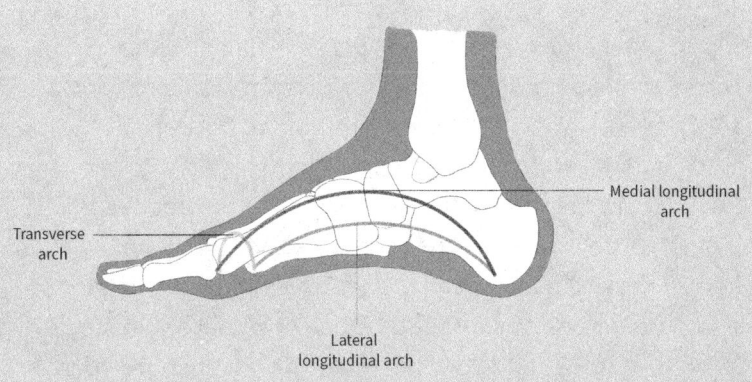

Transverse arch

Medial longitudinal arch

Lateral longitudinal arch

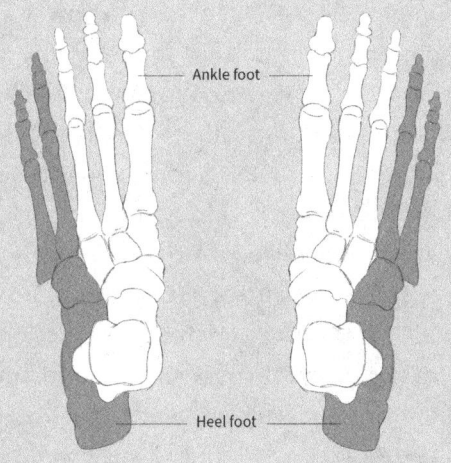

Ankle foot

Heel foot

propulsion, and the heel foot, which is more involved in fine articulation and balance. Your feet really are the most incredible complex piece of engineering!

Now that we have explored the anatomy of the feet, I invite you to explore how it feels to stand with your feet connected to the ground beneath you. Is your weight spread evenly across the anchoring points of your feet, the big toe, the little toe, and the heel? Even just balancing our weight across our feet can transform our posture and make us feel more connected through our bodies.

You might want to explore shifting the weight to see how it feels: leaning forward so that your toes bear your weight, or rocking back to feel the weight in your heels. You might also explore shifting your weight to the inner and outer edges of your feet. Notice how these shifts feel in both your feet and your body, and how it changes your posture. When you come back to the center, spreading your weight evenly across the feet, notice how this allows you to feel more anchored, so that you can grow taller through your body and prepare to focus on the exercise.

Walking barefoot on grass offers more than just a sensory delight; it can positively impact your physical and mental well-being. Walking barefoot helps you to find a connection with nature, while looking out allows you to send your gaze to the horizon or the greenery around you, soothing you, calming your mind, reducing tension, and allowing the level of endorphins (the feel-good hormones) in your body to increase. Walking barefoot can lead to reduced stress, better circulation, and improved sleep. Can you believe that walking barefoot on grass helps you reduce your stress levels by up to 62 percent?[14]

- Find a place in nature that is suitable for walking barefoot: your yard, a park, woods, or a beach. If you can, make sure the area is free from pesticides or herbicides to the best of your knowledge.

- Watch out for sharp objects like stones.

- Generally, start with shorter walks, and gradually build the time spent grounding and allowing your body to adjust.

- Be aware of the temperature. If it is really chilly, be mindful of engaging in a shorter walk so as not to get too cold.

- As you are walking, bring your attention and awareness to your connection with the ground and how the arches and divisions of your feet are working together to support you.

- When you have completed your walk, come to stillness and close your eyes for a moment, reflecting on the sensations in your feet and the groundedness in your body.

- It is good to have tissues or a towel with you to clean your feet before putting your socks and shoes back on.

- Enjoy the sensation of your feet feeling alive and tingling once back inside your shoes.

- Enjoy taking the feeling of the connection with nature with you as you carry on with your day.

FOOT MASSAGE

Now that we have explored the connection of our feet to the earth while walking, I would love to invite you to bring even more awareness to your feet with a foot massage. I hope you'll be surprised and delighted by how this beautiful massage makes your feet feel. It can be done on yourself, or you can work with a partner massaging your feet, which is a beautiful gift to receive as you relax and allow yourself to receive the gift of touch.

At one point in my career, in between dancing and acting, I was intending to work as an alternative therapist. I had learned holistic massage, on-site massage, Jin Shin Jyutsu, and reflexology. I trained in reflexology with the marvelous practitioner Renée Tanner. A foot massage is a fabulous way of releasing tension and grounding yourself, and massaging the feet allows you to connect with every part of your body as your feet are a reflection of the whole of the body. In the end, I did not pursue a career as an alternative therapist, but as part of my work as a movement teacher, my colleague Debbie Green and I conducted an investigation into the training of the feet for actors called "From Grounded Foot to Leaping Foot." Part of this development of work included massaging the feet with techniques taken from Andrea Olsen's *BodyStories*, reflexology techniques taught by Renée Tanner, and techniques shared by Debbie Green.

When I have shared this exercise with students, it is always a joy to feel the profound difference of both groundedness and posture, with just a five-minute massage on each foot. It makes you feel like you're walking on clouds!

In reflexology, each part of the foot links to a different part of the body, as you'll see in the diagram below. This means that massaging the feet also relaxes other parts of the body too.

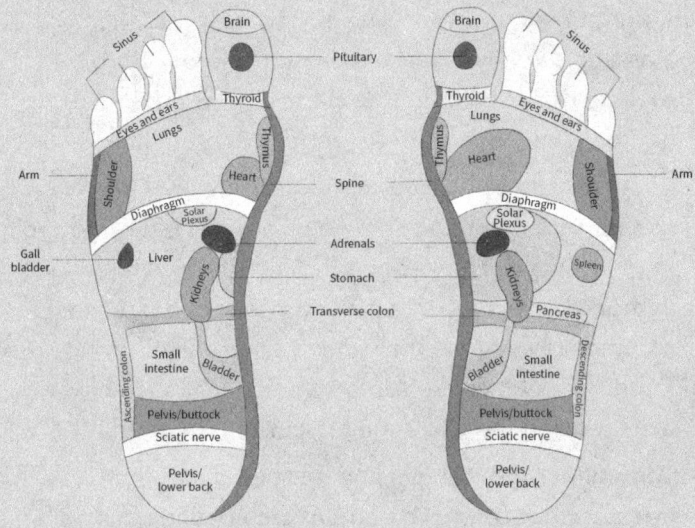

Massaging the right foot

- First, take hold of your right foot with both hands.

- Begin by kneading the foot, as though it were a beautiful piece of dough. Be quite firm as you move your hands down your foot, kneading the ankle and down around the heel. Work across both the top and underside of your foot with this kneading action. Imagine you are saying hello to the whole of the foot.

- As you do this, notice the sensations: Where feels warm and where feels cold? Where feels soft and where feels firmer? Are there any places where you can feel tension?

- Next, bring your attention to the toes. Place your right heel on your left thigh, holding your right foot with your right hand. Your right hand is supporting the weight of your foot so that you can relax into the massage. With your left hand, take hold of your big toe and notice how the toe starts right down in the big toe joint. Your toes are longer than you think!

- Circle the toe from its joint with the head of its metatarsal bone, like stirring a spoon in a bowl, moving it gently in a circular motion through the natural range of motion in the joint. Stir four times in one direction and then reverse the movement, once again stirring four times. Notice the sensations you feel and enjoy experiencing the full range of your toe's motion.

- Throughout this motion, and through the entire massage, notice your breath. Avoid holding your breath, and keep inhaling through the nose and exhaling through your mouth, so that you're releasing your breath all the time.

- Move to your second toe and again notice the length of your toe, all the way to the joint, stirring the toe four times one way and then the other. Continue with each of your toes.

- Once you have finished stirring each toe, spread the toes apart with your hands. Enjoy the "zing" you feel in the webbing between each toe as you give them a beautiful stretch.

- Next, we'll do what I call the caterpillar walk. Spread your big and second toe, and use your index finger to find the channel between the tarsal bones in your feet. Inch your index finger down this channel, as though you were a caterpillar walking down the foot, until the tarsal bones meet at the joint and the finger can go no farther. Focus on spreading the bone, giving space and opening out the muscle. Work along all four spaces between the metatarsal bones.

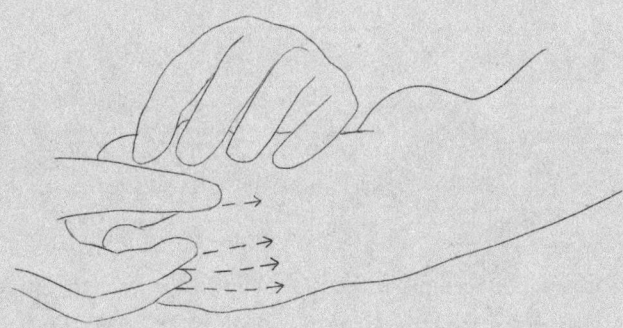

- Notice the sensations between your toes as you do this. Perhaps you might find some points of tension that you can dissipate.

- Notice how the sensation differs in each part of the foot. As mentioned, each part of the foot links to a different part of the body. The top of the foot in this area represents the chest.

- Placing the foot on the floor, continue massaging around the arch of the foot, focusing on moving the skin over the bones, feeling the rise of the arch and the joints between the bones, finally massaging around the line of the ankle.

- With both hands massage around the ankle area.

- Next, with your left hand on your right ankle, with your right hand squeeze behind the ankle, around the Achilles, and journey up the back of the ankle and calf, with gentle squeezes all the way up to behind the knee, and repeat a second time.

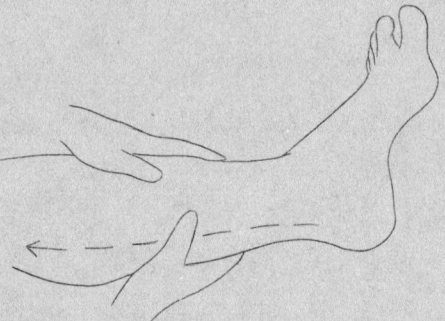

- Once you've finished squeezing all the way up, take your right foot back in your right hand and take hold of the ankle with your left. Feel the joint of your ankle and gently move through the natural rotation of the joint, stirring your ankle like you did for your toes, four times in each direction.

- Then point your toes and stretch down the ankle toward the back of your leg. Enjoy this lovely stretch.

- Reverse this stretch, flexing your toes up, holding on to the heel as you do.

- Alternating between pointing and flexing your foot, enjoy the full range of motion that your ankle is capable of.

- The next part of the massage is called a zigzag. Place your right heel on your left thigh. Position your left hand on the outer edge by the little toe, and your right hand on the inner edge by the big toe. Gently zigzag the foot, stretching the big toe back and little toe forward, then reversing. Continue this zigzagging motion down the instep to the heel. Repeat the sequence once more.

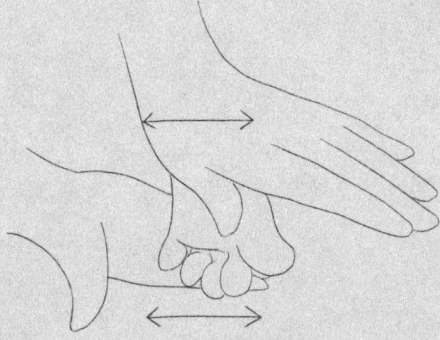

- Next, with your left hand supporting your right foot, fold the fingers of your right hand so you can use the knuckle. Run the knuckle gently down your foot, starting at the big toe, following the instep all the way to the heel. Repeat this once more.

- Then switch hands, supporting your right foot with your right hand. Using the thumb of your left hand, stroke down the outer edge of the foot, from the little toe to the heel. Repeat this movement a second time for balance and release.

- Next, you are going to spread open the four layers of tendons and muscles underneath the foot. Place your thumbs just underneath your toes, across the ball of your feet. And then firmly slide them outward, stretching out the ball of your foot as wide as it can comfortably go.

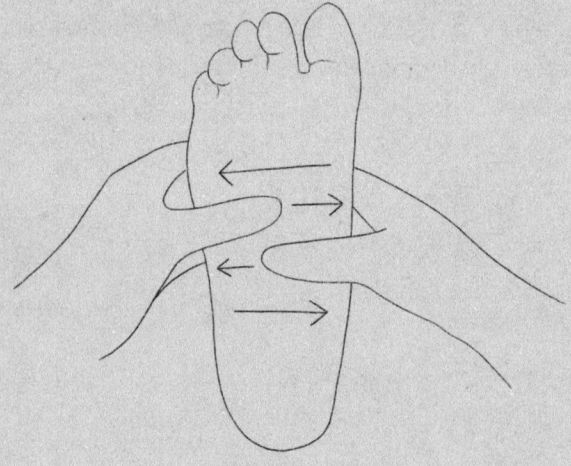

- Gradually make your way down the sole of the foot, stretching out with your thumbs across the ball of the foot, the center of the foot, the height of the instep, and across the heel of the foot right across the entirety of the underside of the foot. Repeat this twice.

- Then place both your thumbs at the center of your heel and draw them up the midline of your foot and, as you get to your toes, spread your foot open, opening the toes out beautifully wide.

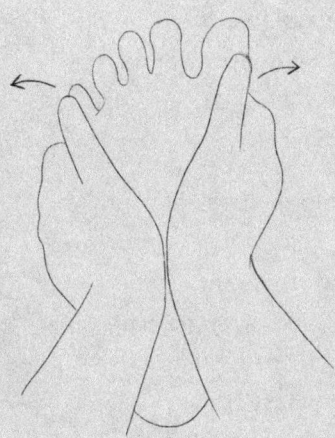

- Next, we find the line that links to the diaphragm. Place your right thumb just below the ball of your foot below the big toe joint, hooking it under the flesh of the ball of your foot.

- Do a caterpillar walk with your thumb along the diaphragm line from under the big toe joint, across to under the little toe joint.

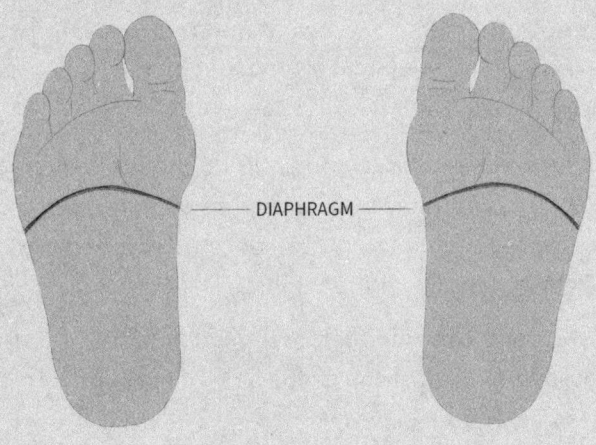

—— DIAPHRAGM ——

- Repeat this walk across the foot, remembering to inhale and exhale deeply as you do.

- Next, bring your thumb back to the midpoint of that line.

- While supporting the back of your foot with your fingers, press your thumb into that midpoint, also known as the bubbling well point, or kidney point 1, continuing to take slow and easy breaths in through your nose and out through your mouth.

- To finish the massage, gently sweep your hands up and off the foot, from ankle to toes, and shake the hands to release any "excess energy."

Feeling the effects of the foot massage

- And now, to understand how that massage might have changed the sensation in your feet, let's take a standing stretch.

- Placing both feet hip-width apart on the ground, come to a ball over the feet. Lift the pelvis so that you hang over the legs, allowing the knees to be soft and the belly to connect with the thighs.

- As you hang over the feet, feel the difference of the release in the hamstring of the side of the foot you have massaged.

- Rolling up through the spine, observe the tensions and stance of the two sides of the body and the connection with the floor of the foot that has been massaged as opposed to the foot that is still to be massaged.

- Feel the line of the buttocks and the shoulder of both sides of the body as you come to standing.

- You can even take a little walk, observing the connection with the floor with both feet, noticing how different both feet might feel from each other now that one has been massaged.

Massaging the left foot

Now to massage the other foot. Repeat the steps for the left foot, switching the instructions for the right hand and foot to the left hand and foot.

To finish:

- Now both your feet have had a beautiful massage, let's take a standing stretch again.

- Placing both feet on the ground, come to a ball over the feet. Lift the pelvis so that you hang over the legs, allowing the knees to be soft and the belly to connect with the thighs, and feel the release in the hamstrings on both legs.

- Rolling up through the spine to a standing position, observe the tensions and stance of the two sides of the body, observing the connection to the floor with both feet.

- Does your connection to the earth feel different now that both feet have been massaged?

- Take a walk again, noticing how the sensations have shifted now that you have explored both feet.

- I hope you'll feel the wonderful articulation through your whole foot, and you may even feel that any tension in your legs, especially your hamstrings, has now dissipated. Enjoy feeling this beautiful new connection from your body through your feet and into the earth.

CHAPTER FOUR

SEEING OURSELVES

One of the biggest barriers we experience in trying to open ourselves to intimacy lies in how we see ourselves, and our relationship with our bodies. In February 2022, Emma Thompson was sitting in front of a roomful of journalists at the Berlin Film Festival when she was asked about a key scene in the film *Good Luck to You, Leo Grande.* In the scene, Thompson's character, Nancy, stands, unmoving, in front of a mirror and looks at her naked body. With startling frankness, Thompson spoke to the journalists about the challenge of delivering an "untreated body" in a film.

"It was hard . . . We're only used to seeing bodies that have, you know, been trained . . . I knew that Nancy wouldn't go to the gym. She would have a normal body of a 62-year-old woman who's had two children. I can't stand in front of a mirror like that. If I stand in front of a mirror, I'll always pull something in . . . I can't just stand there. Why would I do that? It's horrifying. But that's the problem, isn't it?

"Women have been brainwashed all our lives. That's the fact of it. And everything that surrounds us reminds us how imperfect we are and how everything is wrong."[1]

Thompson absolutely puts her finger on something that affects most women—and an increasing number of men. So many of us are unhappy with our bodies, seeing only our faults and imperfections, feeling a kind of embarrassment that we don't look as we dream of looking.

In another interview with *Harper's*, she said something slightly different. "I don't think mirrors are the best invention. They're hard, shiny surfaces reflecting a hard shiny version of the self, and actually they are very good things to cover up from time to time and forget about so that you can re-enter your body and be inside it. We talk about the male gaze and the female gaze and objectification, but we objectify ourselves every time we look in a mirror."[2]

The danger is that those reflecting surfaces do not always represent the truth of who you are, how you feel. That "hard shininess" Thompson references acts as a barrier to intimacy. If you're worried about pulling in your stomach all the time, it is hard to relax into a relationship. If you're concerned that your mascara will smudge, it is difficult to feel and to be passionate. In this chapter we will explore re-entering our bodies, to feel ourselves rather than see ourselves.

In my own life, I have learned to make that shift. I began my career as a dancer, where the image you see in the mirror in front of you is never perfect. There was always further you could go to improve an arabesque, or your line, or a jump. The reflection you saw looking back at you was always a disappointment. As an actor, I realized that the inner voice to be aware of is not the one saying, "I am wrong, I can do better," but the one that questions if you are in your truth and believable. The mirrors are covered in an acting class; you look inward to find emotional connection and impulse, and then communicate that through your voice and your body. It is a fundamental shift.

Seeing ourselves truthfully, finding a real connection with our bodies, is made all the more difficult by the images we see around us. The pictures on our screens—on our phones, in the cinemas, on our TVs—are working as distorting mirrors, showing us false pictures, reflecting not reality but images of unbelievable and unattainable perfection.

I sometimes think about the moment in the Richard Curtis film *Notting Hill* where Julia Roberts's character, Anna Scott, is talking about her life as a film star. She says, "I've been on a diet every day since I was nineteen, which basically means I've been hungry for a decade . . . and it's taken two rather painful operations to get me looking like this . . . And, one day not long from now, my looks will go, they will discover I can't act, and I will become some sad middle-aged woman who looks a bit like someone who was famous for a while."

The speech comes in the middle of a funny scene in a romantic comedy when Roberts is grappling with potential boyfriend William (Hugh Grant) over who gets to eat the last chocolate brownie at dinner. Yet it rings with absolute truth. Ever since Hollywood began to turn normal women into screen goddesses, the effect has been to create an image of womankind that is not just unreal but almost unattainable.

Down the years, there are countless examples of women who have starved and carved themselves into an ideal— often dictated by a man—which has then been held up for other women to follow. Marlene Dietrich is believed to have had teeth removed to give her cheekbones the required shape; Jean Harlow lost her hair thanks to dyeing it with peroxide. In more modern times, many stars openly admit to using Botox, fillers, and other artificial aids to preserve their looks. Still more don't acknowledge the work they are having done to keep up appearances.

Exactly what we value in beauty changes over time, but the Hollywood dream factory always exerts its hold in Western culture, whether it is the thin body of the flappers, or the wasp waists of the '30s, or the more muscular bodies that became popular in the '80s and '90s. When I was starting out as a dancer in the 1970s, the group in vogue were Pan's People; by the time I had left dancing, their lithe bodies had been replaced by those of the more athletic and more overtly sexy Hot Gossip as the appeal of the gym, advertised by stars such as Jane Fonda, began to exert its hold.

The trend of extreme thinness rarely goes away. Beauty standards in celebrity culture have historically and continuously championed thinness as an ideal concept of beauty. When people meet actors in the flesh, they are always surprised by how tiny they are. The well-known adage that the camera adds a dress size means that even women who look relatively average onscreen are often only a UK size 10 (US size 6) or below. Of course, for all its occasional attempts to celebrate plus-size bodies, most of the fashion industry promotes clothes that fetishize the skinny.

Nowhere is this more in evidence than on the red carpet, where the emergence and use of weight-loss drugs such as Ozempic has reintroduced the fashion for extreme thinness. For example, during the 2025 SAG Awards, there was great concern about the skinniness of many of the celebrities posing for photographs. Many of them, both men and women, enjoy the creative expression of how they present themselves, working with their stylists, fashion houses, and their hair and makeup team, to support them in the creation of their image. However, as *Glamour* magazine pointed out, "for many celebrities, weight loss is not just a personal choice, but a professional necessity."[3]

When I worked with Florence Pugh on *We Live in Time*, a love story written by Nick Payne and directed by John Crowley, I was struck by her energy and the robustness in her body. She is brave in all her choices and has spoken brilliantly about her refusal to be defined by other people's expectations of how women should look. She told *ELLE* magazine in an interview with Jodie Turner-Smith in August 2023: "I speak the way I do about my body because I am not trying to hide the cellulite on my thigh or the squidge in between my arm and my boob: I would much rather lay it all out. I think the scariest thing for me are the instances where people have been upset that I've shown 'too much' of myself"—for example, when she chose a see-through pink Valentino dress.

"It's the freedom that people are scared of; the fact I'm comfortable and happy. Keeping women down by commenting on their bodies has worked for a very long time. I think we're in this swing now where lots of people are saying, 'I don't give a shit.' Unfortunately, we've become so terrified of the human body that we can't even look at my two little cute nipples behind fabric in a way that isn't sexual. We need to keep reminding everybody that there is more than one reason for women's bodies to exist."[4]

Amen to that. Lithe, healthy bodies are to be celebrated, as are revealing, beautiful frocks. When we worked together, Pugh shaved her head to play a woman undergoing cancer treatment. She is utterly fearless and without vanity. "Whenever I've not needed to be glam or have a full face of makeup, I fight to keep it that way. It helps the audience," she said.[5]

I entirely agree. On the red carpet, she is consciously sculpting a positive depiction of how she presents herself. Rather than being dictated to, she makes choices using color and a sense of fun that give her an embodied power.

She is deliberately challenging what Emma Thompson so eloquently describes—the way we are brainwashed into accepting just one kind of beauty. Effectively we are being made culturally dysmorphic by the images we see. The American beauty brand Dove has famously built its advertising campaigns around "real women" and in 2004 launched the Dove Self-Esteem Project, which aims by 2030 to have reached half a billion young people with its educational programs.

When it first launched these campaigns, it commissioned a research project that showed a staggering level of unhappiness from women with their looks. Surveying 3,200 women aged between 18 and 24 in 10 countries, it discovered that only 2 percent chose "beautiful" to describe their appearance. Only 9 percent chose "attractive," 8 percent "feminine," 7 percent "good-looking" or "cute."[6] A follow-up experiment, two years later, revealed at least part of the problem: It contrasted photographs of real women with the images that had been airbrushed and manipulated into the advertising photographs that would traditionally be seen on billboards.

A once-ordinary and attractive woman becomes a distorted image: her neck is lengthened, her eyes enlarged, her face slimmed. Yet that is the image that consistently would be sent out into the world and seen as "real," as something we should all aspire to.

The Dove experiment happened way back in 2004. Nowadays, every young woman who wants to alter her appearance doesn't even need the help of an airbrusher or a plastic surgeon. She can simply use the beauty filter that is available on any mobile phone and Photoshop herself into what she perceives as an ideal form. Filters can widen eyes, plump up lips, change the shape of the face. The person who appears on social media can be quite different in appearance from the person who you might meet walking down a street.

This is concerning and has an impact on people of all ages. No wonder we are seeing a significant rise in anxiety and eating disorders among young people. A report published by the Children's Commissioner in the UK in August 2023 estimated that there were 1.25 million people in the UK with eating disorders, and a disproportionate number were below the age of 25. NHS figures for hospital admissions for those suffering from disorders such as anorexia and bulimia rose from 13,200 in 2015–16 to 24,300 in 2020–21. Of those, almost half (11,700) were under the age of 25. While the majority (10,800) were women and girls, admissions of young men had also doubled in that time frame from a smaller base.[7]

I had already been bothered, as I brought up my two children, by noticing how young girls were increasingly unwilling to face the world without makeup. Some of the teenagers I knew would go to bed with their boyfriends wearing full makeup. As beauty editor Loni Venti said in a *Cosmopolitan* article: "I wasn't sure that I could be fun, confident, sexy, smart or the person I wanted to be around him [my boyfriend] without my makeup flawlessly applied."[8] Yet, for intimacy to flourish, for relationships to grow, it requires a journey "into-me-seeing," a level of openness, honesty, and vulnerability between two people. It has been so refreshing to see Pamela Anderson, who found fame as a highly made-up *Baywatch* beauty, championing a "no makeup" look, embracing her natural loveliness and looking as gorgeous as she has ever been. In a *Guardian* interview she explained: "I spent some time for myself, stripping away this caricature that I created, because I'd started believing that it was true. You have to have self-acceptance."[9]

However, in television and on film, women nearly always go to bed in full makeup and wake up the same way. It is still rare to see a woman take off her makeup on film.

When I go to work now, I quite deliberately don't wear makeup. I'd wear makeup to go on stage, or if I was going out. But when I am being creative, making work with others, I want to be present to others and present in my work. I want to be utterly myself to make it as easy as possible for people to interact with me; elaborate makeup, worn all the time, is just another barrier we put in place between ourselves and the world.

Alongside the literally distorting effects of technology are the insidious and equally alarming effects of social media in general. In 2022, I worked on the sci-fi series *The Peripheral* with Chloë Grace Moretz, an actress who has the ability to embody a character in a profound and detailed way. Since I worked with her, Moretz has revealed that the widespread internet sharing of a meme based on a photograph taken in New York in 2016 that turned her into a character from *Family Guy,* with very long legs and a short torso, had caused her to become a virtual recluse. "To this day, when I see that meme, it's something very hard for me to overcome," she said. "I think that body dysmorphia—which we all deal with in this world—is extrapolated by issues of social media. It's a headfuck."[10]

What happened to Moretz, as a celebrity, happens to so many of our teenagers every day. Pictures of their bodies, dressed and sometimes undressed, are shared and discussed by their peers, with and without their consent. Not only that, immature and uncertain youngsters are being bombarded with harmful content by algorithms that serve to increase their anxieties and that actually target the most vulnerable. Research in 2023 revealed that TikTok accounts registered for 13-year-olds were being shown videos advertising weight-loss drinks and "tummy tuck" surgery. Videos relating to body image, mental health, and eating disorders were shown to "vulnerable" accounts three times more than to standard accounts.[11]

It is still mainly women and girls who are most subject to this level of body shaming and anxiety. But our boys and young men are increasingly feeling pressured too. Traditionally, men have been allowed to grow old onscreen, to get older, more rugged, more husky and craggy, and be celebrated for that, while the women they act opposite get ever younger. This has trapped women in a cycle of endless youth. You only had to watch the *Friends* reunion in 2021 to see this. All the women looked pretty much as they did 20 years ago, while the men were quite different, graying, carrying more weight. But recently, it seems to me that male actors too feel they can only be seen on film with ripped muscles and six-packs.

I was conscious of this when I was working on *Magic Mike's Last Dance,* the third film about a group of male strippers, a film that in many ways is incredibly positive in the kind of sexuality it puts onscreen. It shows consent in action, with women being put in the position where they can choose the kind of closeness and intimacy that they enjoy. It also, in the shape of Salma Hayek, offers an inspiring vision of a woman who pays attention to her sexual needs.

But the film's star, Channing Tatum, made a very interesting observation about the discipline it had taken him to sculpt his body in this way. Talking on *The Kelly Clarkson Show,* he said that the way his body looked onscreen went beyond a healthy, consistent workout routine. "It's hard even if you work out to be in that kind of shape," he said, adding that it wasn't a question of eating well. He wouldn't even use that word. "That's not even healthy. You have to starve yourself. I don't think when you're that lean, it's actually healthy for you."[12]

In order to look toned in this way onstage or on film, the performers follow a regime of nutrition that involves them timing when they eat carbohydrates and protein, so they will build muscle, and the body looks very lean and the muscles are defined. Sometimes they stop drinking water, even when they are dancing energetically.

When he was filming a topless scene in *The Batman,* Robert Pattinson admitted that he virtually stopped drinking water because he wanted to look his best. Speaking to *People* magazine in 2022, he said he had worked on his appearance for about three months before filming started, "and then you are working out before and after work all the time. You just cut down, and cut down, and cut down before the couple of scenes with your shirt off, and you're counting sips of water."[13]

This is a regime that can be maintained only for a short amount of time—and yet somehow it is being presented as an image to aspire to. It isn't natural, and it isn't normal. People can't live like that. It's got very little to do with a healthy lifestyle of eating well and doing good exercise. Like so much of what we see onscreen, it is an illusion—but it is an image people feel they have to match in real life. There is a pushback going on, to try to break the cycle. It is really positive when someone like Channing Tatum or Robert Pattinson speaks out and explains what it involves. It is not that everyone onscreen should be overweight or unmuscular, but it is important to explain that this is not an attainable way to look in real life.

Yet the pressures of social media can make people feel they should. In my work, I've come across actors who start to fear leaving the house in case the paparazzi—or just someone with a camera phone—snaps them looking less than perfect. It breaks my heart. They are handsome, healthy actors, yet they feel they are not "ripped," with a perfectly defined six-pack. That obsession is stopping them being themselves, inhibiting their ability to be free and open. It is exactly what female actors have suffered for so many years.

Kate Winslet, whose appearance has been the subject of so much comment since she first appeared onscreen, has always taken a stand against women being "bullied" about their appearance. Talking to the *Happy Sad Confused* podcast, to mark the twenty-fifth anniversary of her breakthrough film, *Titanic*, she took to task journalists and fans who said she was fat. "Why were they so mean to me? I wasn't even fat. I would have said to journalists . . . 'Don't you dare treat me like this. I'm a young woman, my body is changing, I'm figuring it out, I'm deeply insecure, I'm terrified, don't make this any harder than it already is.' That's bullying, you know, and actually borderline abusive I would say."[14]

As she established herself as a power within the film industry, Winslet has used her influence to change things. At the age of 27, she took *GQ* magazine to task for airbrushing a cover image of her. "I do not look like that, and more importantly, I don't have a desire to look like that," she said.[15] When she was making the television series *Mare of Easttown,* some eighteen years later at the age of 45, she refused to let the director hide what Hollywood calls physical "imperfections." She wouldn't approve the show's promotional poster until the airbrushing on her face had been removed and she would not allow the director Craig Zobel to cut "a bulgy bit of belly" that was shown in an intimate scene with her co-star Guy Pearce. She told him "Don't you dare!"

In an interview with *The New York Times*, she said: "I hope that in playing Mare as a middle-aged woman—I will be 46 in October—I guess that's why people have connected with this character in the way that they have done because there are clearly no filters. She's a fully functioning, flawed woman with a body and a face that moves in a way that is synonymous with her age and her life and where she comes from. I think we're starved of that a bit."[16]

I agree. I have worked on a couple of occasions (on *Sex*

Education and *Bad Sisters*) with Anne-Marie Duff, who told me that women actually come up to her on the street and thank her for resisting the pressure to alter her appearance with any kind of plastic surgery. Duff is a beautiful woman who, in her words, is not "Botoxed up to the nines." "I made that decision, and some people think it's bonkers . . . It's such an emotive thing, you know?"[17]

Frances McDormand is another role model for women who aren't afraid to age. Now in her sixties, she has been vocal against plastic surgery—rejecting Botox, fillers, hair dye, and quite often, makeup, even when accepting her second, third, and fourth Oscars for *Three Billboards Outside Ebbing, Missouri* in 2018 and for *Nomadland* in 2021. Women are made to feel aging is their problem, she says, but it's a cultural problem, not a personal one. All of us will age, after all. If we are lucky.

"Getting older and adjusting to all the things that biologically happen to you is not easy to do, and is a constant struggle and adjustment," she said, emphasizing her belief that cosmetic surgery and enhancement make it harder, not easier. "I think it makes it much more difficult to accept getting older. I want to be revered. I want to be an elder; I want to be an elderess."[18]

McDormand, Pugh, Duff, Winslet, and women like them are part of an informal campaign against false impressions and for wanting to present more reality in what we see. Winslet made a TV program, *I Am Ruth,* with her daughter Mia Threapleton about the relationship between a mother and her closed-off teenage daughter who is increasingly consumed by the pressures of social media, taking desperate selfies, hiding under her duvet as notifications pile up. "It can be extremely negative," she said at the time. "People are subject to scrutiny that is more than a young, vulnerable person can cope with."[19]

It is definitely true in my experience that change is underway. But it is sometimes held back by a reluctance on the part of some producers to let actors be real onscreen. On at least three occasions in my experience as an intimacy coordinator, female actors have refused to remove their body hair; on each occasion there has been considerable pushback to make them wax or shave. When one actor stood her ground, her scenes were filmed with her character wearing her stockings. No hair was ever seen onscreen. Body hair for men is becoming equally unseen. Just compare Sean Connery's James Bond, with his naturally hairy chest in the 1960s, with Daniel Craig's virtually hairless body forty-five years later.

Yet body hair is part of life, part of our relationship with our bodies. It's the same with menstruation. Fifty percent of the world's population menstruate for, on average, forty years of their life for about a week every month. Therefore, half of the world's population, for around 480 weeks during their lives, are engaged in the paraphernalia of menstruation: tampons, menstrual cups, period pads, and painkillers! Yet how often do you see that onscreen? Even on advertisements that were selling us sanitary products, for years advertisers were too embarrassed to make the liquid poured into the absorbent pad a color other than blue. Only recently has any red liquid appeared.

One way in which Michaela Coel's *I May Destroy You* was so groundbreaking was that it not only showed a woman having sex while on her period, but it actually showed her partner taking the tampon out and the resulting blood clot. I supported the choreography of that scene, making sure every beat of the process was registered. The truthfulness shone through. Michaela's writing made it clear that there was no sense of disgust: the man's reaction was one of pleasure and discovery, examining the clot and describing its beauty.

This marked such a change from the denial about menstrual bodily functions that are rarely seen in our stories in TV, film, and theater. It's important that the narratives we see include realistic depictions of women's experiences in life. It's all part of acknowledging that the images we are bombarded by are false and unhelpful. Seeing ourselves truthfully involves a confidence in knowing that we don't have to conform and learning to cultivate a positive dialogue with our bodies and ourselves.

In my experience, actors sometimes fear the changing room, where they have to encounter the difference between the self as it is and the character they are about to play, as they are fitted for their costumes and come face to face with the image they will present on stage or onscreen. They are navigating the space between their personal self and their professional self and have to navigate the physical transformation from their experience of themselves and their relationship to their body to the physicality they are offering of themselves in service of the character. Vulnerabilities emerge in the gulf between how they see themselves and how they want to present themselves to the world at large.

Feeling discontent and unhappy with our body image traps us in a metaphorical changing room, lacking the confidence to believe that our body, as it is, can be attractive in relationships. If society is telling us that we should look certain ways to which we don't conform, then we are trying to fit ourselves into costumes and masks. The lesson we can take is to try to avoid being forced into a corset of someone else's making and allow ourselves to be who we want to be.

The way out is to work on our connection with ourselves and our bodies, and through that find a new self-assurance. Part of being confident in our bodies is about nurturing our sense of awareness of our corporeal selves and who we are.

When I teach Body-Mind Centering (BMC), I realize that it creates an incredible appreciation of our bodies and their functions. BMC is described as an embodied approach to movement, body, and one's consciousness. This physical exploration was developed by Bonnie Bainbridge Cohen, a most wonderful human being who is "a movement artist, researcher, educator, and therapist, and the developer of the BMC approach to movement, the body, and consciousness." I had the joy of attending a week-long course with Bainbridge Cohen in June 2011. It is the closest I have come to being in the presence of a living master, and it was such a privilege to learn from Bonnie in the room.

Exploring yourself within all the structures of your physicality, you explore the bone structure, the skeleton, the muscles, the journey of the nervous system through your body. You explore the organs in sounding and in movement, of the lungs; the digestive system; the qualities of the liver, pancreas, and spleen; the cleansing power of the urinary tract and the kidneys; and the reproductive energy of the sexual organs, the womb, and the gonads.

When you get to the heart, you feel its electrical energy keeping the body alive, the arterial flow going out into the world and the venous flow of energy back into the heart. When you meet someone, you are responding unconsciously to that energy. If you feel it consciously, suddenly you are perceiving your body in quite a different way, not as something that you look at in a mirror but as a living, breathing, powerful entity that connects you to the world.

When I used to teach students, I asked them to work in pairs and experience the bones through the touch of their partner, letting them feel the shapes beneath the skin: the long bones running down the arms and legs, metatarsals and phalanges of the feet, and the metacarpals and phalanges of the hand that give your body direction in space, and the curved bones of the skull, ribs, and pelvis protecting your organs.

Then there are the tarsals and carpals, the bones that articulate our feet and hands. I try to get students to feel the articulation of the spine, from the delicate bones of the cervical vertebrae to the thoracic vertebrae, each with a pair of ribs hanging down and around to encase the organs of the thorax. And then go on to feel the lumbar vertebrae, the largest bones of the spine at the center of the body, the fused bones of the sacrum and the fine bones of the coccyx, of the ancestral tail. I might suggest that they roll around on the floor, feeling the elliptical quality of the skull, or the curve of the rib cage and the bowl of the pelvis. It is quite freeing when you are working in this way. The concentration on each area of the bony structure gives you a different experience of yourself in the architecture of the body, and the quality of movement with clear direction and ease through space.

I might spend two to three terms exploring the different organs of the body and the feelings they generate. We might spend time, for example, thinking about the liver, which, after the skin, is the largest organ in the body, and is responsible for over 500 functions. It is the organ of stability, of detoxifying, of dealing with heavy emotions that require processing, such as anger. I invite the students to turn to Shakespeare, who is always referring to the organs, including the liver, and relate their experience of the liver to the delivery of the speech in Shakespeare's *Much Ado About Nothing* where Friar Francis points out that "love—especially passionate love, whose rush cannot be easily controlled—resides in the human liver." Interestingly, in Greek mythology, the liver is regarded as the location of one's passion, emotion, anger, and wrath.

In terms of intimacy, if we are thinking about our body in relation to others, then the key organ is obviously your heart, feeling into its rhythm as the fundamental dynamo of the body. I might ask people to work in pairs—and you can do this with a partner or with a friend—to feel each other's pulse and beat out the rhythm felt on a drum and walk to that rhythm. Everyone's heart has a different quality and a different feeling to it. If you are literally moving to the beat of someone else's heart, then you are moving into a sense of intimacy with them.

Another way in which you can experience the quality of the heart is to try a heart-to-heart dance with your partner. This whole-body connection is truly an intimate thing. A heart dance is an exercise in synchronizing energy. I quite often use it in a rehearsal room when I want to support people who have only just met in becoming comfortable with one another. But, in an intimate setting, it takes on added value. The exercise, which I first came across when partaking in a BMC workshop led by Mark Chandlee Taylor in 2008, consists of creating two circles, an inner and outer circle, where people stand facing one another. If you are doing it with your partner, there are obviously just the two of you. The exercise is as follows:

- Begin by standing with your hands on your own heart, and imagine the space behind it, how it makes you feel about yourself, how you love yourself, how you allow yourself to be loved and the love you have to send out to others in the world.
- You then put your right hands on each other's hearts and your left hands over your partner's hand on your heart, consciously inviting the neurological connection of touch, completing a circle.
- Pause and be fully present, feeling the movement, the energy, and the dance between you. It's a beautiful connection. Close your eyes, and you may be amazed at how much closer it brings you, and how differently it makes you feel.

If you are exploring this exercise by yourself, you can engage in the first part of the exercise, connecting with your own heart, and then have an image of giving love to yourself and taking yourself on a heart dance, following the impulses you feel and the expression of your love for yourself. This is a wonderful and joyful practice where you can indulge in following your impulses and giving yourself exactly what you need, and how you want to express yourself in the moment.

When I am working with a group with inner and outer circles facing each other, as described above, I will ask participants to change partners, so that they get a sense of the variations in energy from each different encounter.

Having the opportunity to connect consciously with different people's heart energy is a profound and beautiful experience.

You can develop the bond by offering to move to a hug, chest to chest, which again enables you to feel the connection with someone's heart. You might breathe into the hug for a few moments. Or you might stay with the hand on your partner's heart being covered by your hand, then close your eyes and begin to move together very slowly, feeling where the heart dance takes you. The connection is utterly lovely because in order to engage, you need to slow down, listen with your body and with your energy. It takes you to a different experience of intimacy that is beyond words, as you fall entirely into sync with another human being.

Unconsciously, of course, we do this all the time when we meet people—we sense their energy and their compatibility with our own feelings. When you meet someone, you talk about just wanting to be around them, or about how you could have talked all night. We stand opposite someone and are naturally drawn to them. But when you do it as a conscious thing, it has an extraordinary effect. According to the HeartMath Institute, the heart's electrical field is about sixty times greater in amplitude than the electrical activity generated by the brain. This field, measured in the form of an electrocardiogram (ECG), can be detected anywhere on the surface of the body.[20] The wonder of feeling someone's heart energy quite often reduces people to tears.

Once you start experiencing your body in this different way, journeying through its richness rather than critically studying it from outside, you are liberating yourself to be yourself, allowing yourself to be who you are rather than who you might think you ought to be.

This is so important in building intimate relations, whether with friends or with partners. The relaxation that comes when you feel comfortable with your physical appearance allows you to embrace your intimate relationships more fully. It enables you to flirt, to enjoy someone else's company, to explore someone else's body without shame or embarrassment.

It's crucial to remember in this context that chemistry between two people isn't really about outer appearance. That counts for something, but it can't count for everything. In auditions in the past, actors have sometimes been asked to kiss so that a casting director can see if there is an attraction between them. This is a misunderstanding of the nature of attraction. Chemistry is not about beauty; it's about connection and spark, the space between.

The movement and acting practitioner Jacques Lecoq encouraged the idea of *le jeu* or play. He invited his students to improvise, to make the most of whatever material was available and bring the moment alive. His ideas are important to me when it comes to building intimacy. In relationships, you want to find those moments when you glance tantalizingly over your shoulder, or flash your eyes, which electrifies the space between you and your partner and creates a bond.

Being able to give and receive love in this way is about loving yourself, accepting yourself, and then looking outward to those you are in a relationship with. It is about extending your charisma out into the world. The people whom we think of as charismatic, whether they are politicians or actors, have a sense of being open to everything, of illuminating the space. Just watching someone like Cate Blanchett, Andrew Scott, or Olivia Colman step into a room, you see the effect. They fill their own kinesphere like a beacon of energy and light. You know you are in the presence of someone who is extraordinary in how they inhabit themselves and the power of who they are.

It's something actors learn to do, and it's something anyone can learn. Actors think about their projection in terms of three circles. The first circle is your relationship with yourself, the second is you in relationship, the third circle is you in relationship with your audience and letting your audience into that bubble. You can see this in action with many performers. In 1984, I went to see Bruce Springsteen perform at Wembley, and when he told anecdotes between the songs, it was as if you were sitting in his living room. In that vast arena, he extended his kinesphere, so it hit the back of the stadium and encompassed everyone in the auditorium. It is an extraordinary skill, but it is one that can help everyone as they build relationships.

(See page 132 for an exercise that will help you explore your kinesphere.)

In terms of seeing ourselves, although I am no expert on the subject, I recognize and welcome that awareness of gender fluidity and gender expression adds another layer to the way many people, young and old, view their bodies. In schools where I have taught and on productions where I have worked, I have noticed not only an increasing acceptance of different gender expression but also support for young people who are changing their gender identity, either by living as a different gender from the one assigned at birth or by transitioning.

We've all come to recognize, as an article in Harvard Health noted, that "for some youth, gender fluidity may be a way to explore gender before landing on a more stable gender expression or identity. For others, gender fluidity may continue indefinitely as part of their life experience with gender . . . Not everyone who experiences changes in their gender expression or identity identifies as gender-fluid. Nor does everyone desire gender-affirming medical treatment to change their body to better align with their gender identity."[21]

Understanding and appreciating all these possibilities about the freedom that comes from feeling connected with your body will become increasingly important moving forward. It's all about having the courage and the sense of self-worth that allows you to feel happy in your own skin and that you have something to offer. This is true in every intimate relationship with our loved ones: with friends, with family, and with our potential or actual partners.

It would help us all to become more comfortable with our own bodies if we saw more bodies of diverse shapes and sizes and their natural functions onscreen. It felt radical when Michaela Coel showed menstruation as a normal part of lovemaking because it was true. I feel that as filmmakers, we have a responsibility to show bodies and lovemaking as they might be in the world rather than through a sanitized lens. We want people to feel they can be sexy without a six-pack and comfortable with their body hair, and to feel that they don't have to conform to an idealized notion of beauty in order to have a satisfactory intimate relationship with a lover.

As I've continued my own exploration of intimacy, I have noticed how people—particular young people—feel they need to shave their pubic hair as soon as they become sexually active. That has become the new normal, and that trend has in turn led to the rise of young women in particular feeling that their newly exposed vulva is somehow abnormal or misshaped. In the absence of positive education on the anatomy of the female, where the spectrum of normal appearance described for the vulva is woefully misunderstood, women are suffering from feeling their vulva is misshapen, ugly, and a source of shame and embarrassment. It's a cycle: Shaving pubic hair (encouraged by pornography and social media) exposes the female genitalia, which in turn places an emphasis on how the genitalia look. This has led to an alarming rise in labiaplasty surgery to reduce the size of the labia minora. Sometimes there are health reasons for reducing the size of the labia, but this rise in labiaplasties is being driven by women, girls, and gender-diverse people wanting to alter the look of their vulva purely for cosmetic reasons.

In a podcast discussion between sexual health educators Nina Brochmann and Ellen Støkken Dahl, who wrote *The Wonder Down Under: A User's Guide to the Vagina*, Brochmann says: "When we learn about puberty at school, we see how the penis grows and changes, but no one really educates us about how female genitals develop or change." Støkken Dahl adds: "The inner labia have a sexual function: they're full of nerve endings and it feels good to touch them." She goes on to say, "My vagina feels good, and that's what sex is about: feeling good. Ultimately, the world makes it hard for us women to love our bodies. Just talking about our vaginas is difficult—but they are wonderful. No two are the same, and there's no such thing as a good one or a bad one. Every vulva and vagina is awesome, and the more we say it out loud, the easier it is to start believing it."[22]

A report published by Women's Health Victoria in Australia in 2024 found that almost a quarter (23 percent) of respondents aged 18 to 24 felt anxious, unhappy, or embarrassed about how their labia look, while 35 percent associate their labia with negative words such as "weird," "disgusting," or "ugly."[23] One in ten of the 1,030 respondents said they had considered labiaplasty. Experts quoted in an article in *Cosmopolitan* magazine point out that, given the diversity in the anatomy of the labia, it's important not to normalize a specific size or shape or for people to try to conform to a single idea of what the labia should look like, as you can see in the wonderful drawings by Hazel Mead on page 126 of vulvas and penises of all shapes and sizes. Indeed, the vulva shape considered to be "the norm," nicknamed the Barbie, with small, closed lips where the labia minora (the inner lips) are hidden by the labia majora (the outer lips), is the least common type of vulva.[24]

I am all in favor of being much more open about this. It is important that we are supported in knowing that everything is normal. The Channel 4 program *Naked Attraction*, in which prospective partners are judged by their nude anatomy, has its detractors; in particular it caused immense controversy when it was streamed in the US, with an article stating, "The full frontal nudity remains a frontier of reality programming that American television, for all its contrivances and trashiness and barrel-scraping, has yet to reach."

But it does have the virtues of frankness and honesty, and above all, it reveals the range and diversity of our bodies. Defending the show to the *Hollywood Reporter*, the executive producer Darrell Olson said it proves "that every person is different, and not just facially. We've all got different genitals. We've all got different big toes. It's amazing. So there's no reason to feel bad about yourself, and it's empowering to see we're all different."[25]

The point is made even more powerfully by a trilogy of books by the author and photographer Laura Dodsworth: *Bare Reality: 100 Women, Their Breasts, Their Stories*; *Manhood: The Bare Reality*; and *Womanhood: The Bare Reality*. In each, she presents images of the nude body—of breasts, penises, and vulvas—alongside text in which the anonymous people photographed talk about how they feel about their bodies.

The cumulative effect is remarkable. It's not just that they celebrate and show all different types of normal, but that they allow their participants—men and women, gay, straight, and trans, of different skin colors and generations—to talk in depth about how we live in our bodies and how we react to the comments and judgments of others.

As she conducted the interviews, Dodsworth discovered how much shame about our bodies can condition the way we feel. Women are turning away from pleasure because they're worried about how they look, smell, and taste. "Shame is a really big problem for human beings," she said in an interview. "Where I've found that, generally, men are under pressure to be 'enough'—big enough, getting laid enough, rich enough, man enough—women feel like they're 'too much'—too fat, too hairy, too saggy, too female. Frankly, we just need to be as we are."[26]

Another positive resource is The Great Wall of Vulva, by the artist Jamie McCartney, which consists of life-sized plaster molds of the genitalia of more than 400 women,

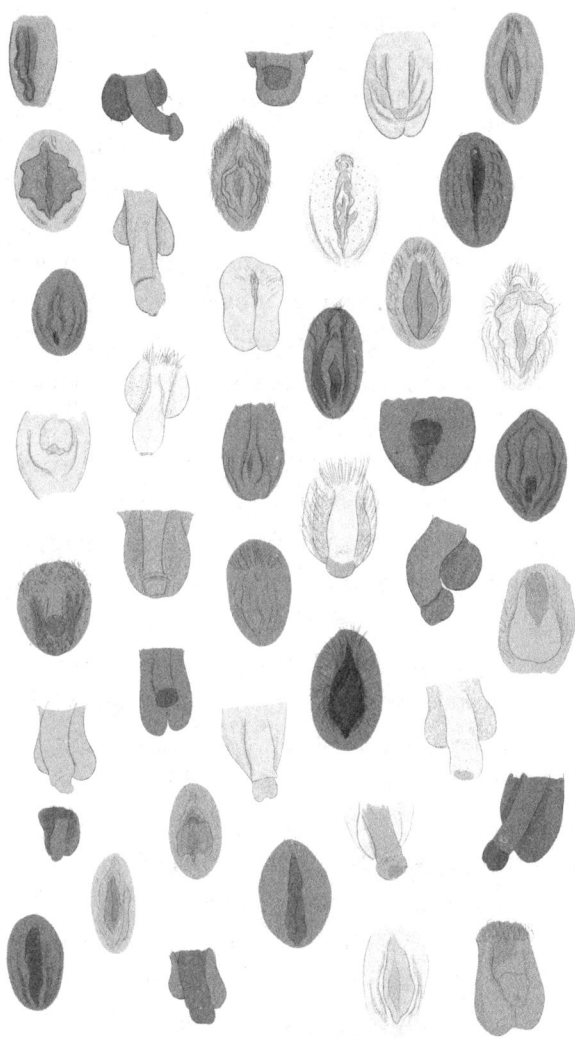

eight meters long, arranged into ten large panels. Being presented in this artistic form offers a more abstracted experience that allows viewers to contemplate the varied beauty of the female form.

What I value in both Dodsworth's and McCartney's work

is the way it seeks to give a positive representation of bodies, of vulva, penis, and breast shapes, that are as individual as a fingerprint. By understanding who we are, by really looking and celebrating, we are creating something richer than the stereotypical images that pornography, social media, and advertising seek to persuade us are the norm. Accepting this about ourselves, be it as a woman, man, nonbinary, or trans person, knowing that what every part of us looks like is not just normal but beautiful, encourages the building of a relationship with the body that is empowering and confident, rather than negative and critical. To appreciate your body for all it does. To love the bits you love, and also to love even more the bits that you don't love!

In her book *Come As You Are*, Emily Nagoski speaks not only about the consequence of women's constant self-criticism and the negative effect this has on our own mental and physical health and well-being, but also how this influences our relationships. "Women who feel worse about their bodies have less satisfying, riskier sex, with less pleasure, more unwanted consequences and more pain," she says.[27]

By working toward being more comfortable with our bodies, seeing ourselves as beautiful, and shifting our approach to living healthily in our bodies, we can use the mirror as our ally. Taking time to be present with your body image and positively focusing on changing the narrative of how you respond to what you see in the mirror is one of the most empowering practices you can engage with in loving yourself. I encourage you to nurture self-love, self-acceptance, and the willingness to embrace the possibility that you are perfect just as you are.

To help you explore this further, I have suggested some exercises (see the following pages).

In my work, I have come to see the beauty of the naked body, in all its shapes and forms, when there is an ease and an honesty from the person displaying it. It is about finding confidence inside ourselves in order to be truly present in our bodies and to take this presence and love of self into our relationships with our loved ones. Self-acceptance and self-love can take us all away from the tyranny of the mirror, with its hard shiny surfaces, and help us move toward engaging with the mirror as our ally and entering a gentler and more intimate space.

The more we can connect to our bodies and treat ourselves with kindness, love, and acceptance, the more we can take this love and relish how we can enjoy and share that love in our relationships and sexual encounters.

MIRROR AFFIRMATIONS

Mirror affirmations, pioneered by Louise Hay in her books *You Can Heal Your Life* and *The Power Is Within You,* are beautiful ways to build confidence and connection with yourself. Using the mirror as an ally, you can truly see and appreciate yourself in all your glory. Below I have suggested three different variations of mirror affirmations, and I invite you to explore them yourself.

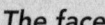

The face

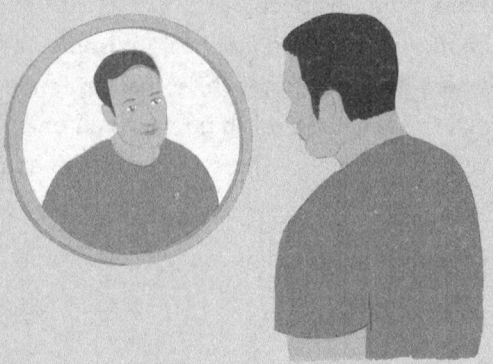

- Find a quiet moment when you will be undisturbed and stand in front of a mirror.

- Look into your own eyes, noticing all that you can see. Maintain eye contact with yourself, connecting with yourself and grounding yourself in this moment.

- Move your gaze slowly across your own face, appreciating the shapes, colors, and textures. Observe yourself without judgment: simply notice what you can see. What do you appreciate about yourself?

- Speak positive affirmations to yourself, maintaining eye contact. You can find the affirmations that inspire and energize you. Some examples might be:

   I love and approve of myself
   I accept myself unconditionally
   I am healthy, whole, and complete just as I am.

- Repeat your affirmation several times and allow yourself to absorb how it feels to treat yourself with kindness, and to express these positive beliefs. Over time, regular mirror affirmations can help your positive beliefs about yourself to overcome any negative beliefs you may be carrying, and to adapt the affirmations to support you with whatever you wish to focus on.

The body

You can also apply mirror affirmations to your whole body.

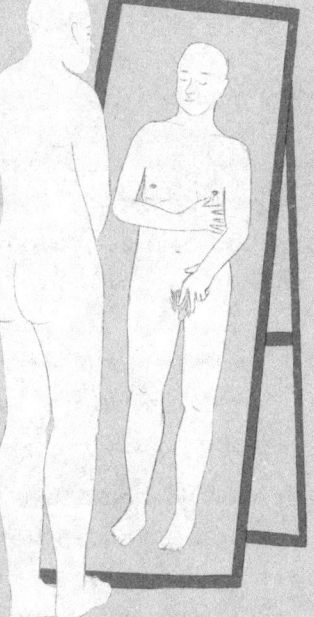

- Find a warm, quiet space where you will be undisturbed. Take off your clothes and stand in front of the mirror.

- Allow your gaze to wander slowly over your whole

body. Notice the areas that you like and appreciate, and take a moment to feel this appreciation for your body. As with the first mirror affirmation, you can say these observations aloud, or you can simply notice them in your mind.

- Now allow yourself to focus on the parts of your body that you find harder to love, or that cultural messages have told you are less valuable. Consider what these parts of the body do for you and what you appreciate about these body parts.

- Take this moment to appreciate what these body parts have given you.

- Express these observations and this gratitude for the power and beauty of your body.

The genitals

We rarely take the time to truly get to know our genitals, especially those with a vulva because it is more hidden in the body. I invite you to take a hand mirror, and to explore and get to know your vulva.

- Find a comfortable position to sit or stand so that you can hold a mirror beneath or beside your vulva and get a good view.

- Allow your gaze to rest on your vulva, observing the shapes, colors, and textures of your unique and beautiful anatomy. Notice the shape of the lips of your labia and of your clitoris. Observe your body hair

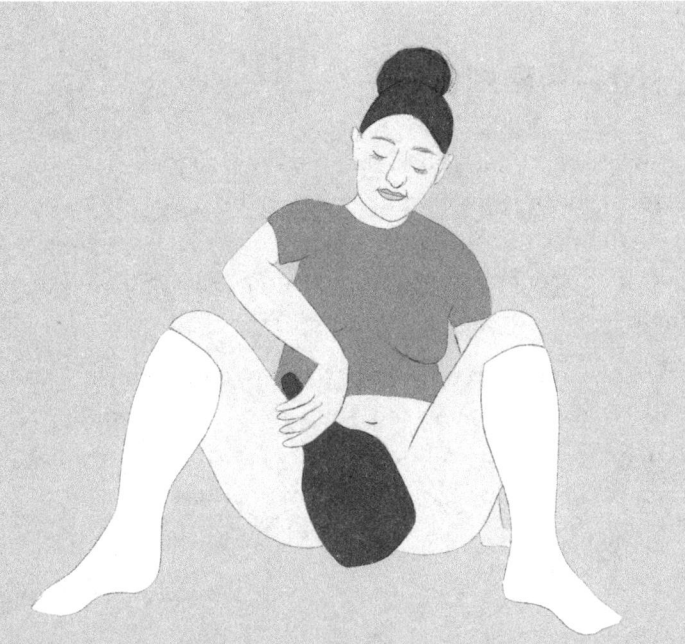

and truly appreciate this place of amazing creativity. If you feel comfortable, express these observations aloud.

- You may also wish to use your free hand to feel your genitals; this can give you an even greater understanding of the shapes, textures, and feelings of this wonderful part of your body.

- Take a moment to express your appreciation for all that you can notice and feel, truly seeing your vulva as it is, in all its unique glory.

    Those with a penis can also explore this exercise by observing their penis and testicles in a mirror, noticing the shapes, textures, and appearance of their genitals.

KINESPHERE

This exercise invites you to explore the boundaries of your personal space, your own energetic bubble. As you stand, take a moment to sense the space around you, noticing how far your energy extends and gently tracing the edges of that invisible boundary.

- Start by reaching up with both arms. Once you've reached as far as you can, snap your fingers and imagine placing a star at the very top of your personal space, at the uppermost edge of your reach.

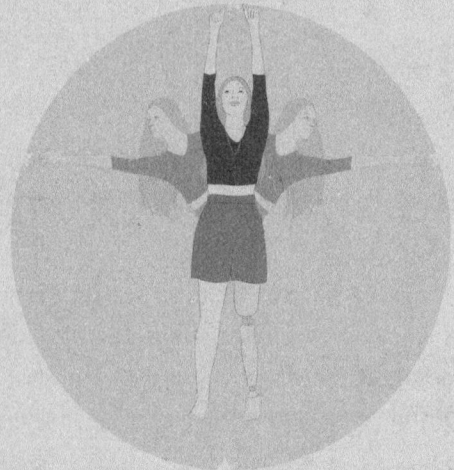

- Enjoy really feeling the height of that space, and then bring your arms back down, imagining that the star has stayed where you left it, hovering above your head.

- Then, do the same for the other edges of your space, beginning with your right side.

- With your right arm, reach out to your right side, as far as you can stretch your arm without moving your feet. When you've extended to the very edge of your reach, click your fingers again, imagining that you're placing that twinkling star at that farthest point to your right. Feel the connection to the swirling stars above your head and to the right side.

- Now repeat this movement with your left arm, reaching as far as you can to the edge of the personal space on your left side, and adding another twinkling star as you click your fingers to the left.

- Staying connected with those twirling stars above your head and to the sides, bring your arms down and reach down past your feet. As you click your fingers here, imagine these twirling stars are hovering at an arm's length into the earth below you.

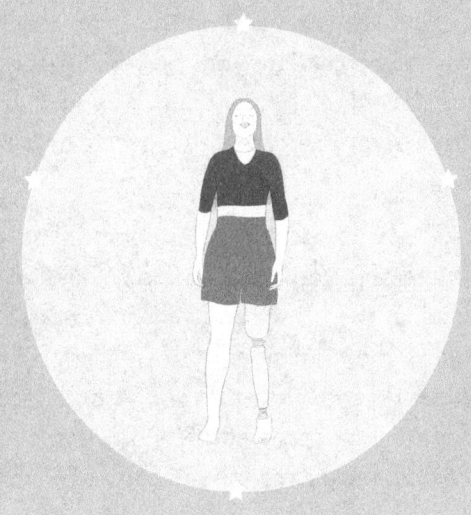

- Come back to standing and take a moment to feel the twirling stars above your head, to the right side of you, to the left side of you, and down below your feet.

- Now bring your arms forward and stretch, reaching straight out in front of you as far as you can, snapping your fingers and placing a new star at the outer point of your arms' reach.

- Feel those wonderful stars and enjoy that space you've claimed for yourself.

- Now, to continue tracing our personal space, it is really important to extend our bubbles behind us too. We very often forget this aspect of our personal space, the part that extends behind us.

- Start with your right hand and reach as far as you can, clicking your fingers to place that star behind you. Come back to the center, remembering the breath.

- Now take your left hand and do the same, reaching back as far as you can into your personal space and clicking to leave that star hovering. As you come back to the center again, feel those stars twinkling around you.

- These stars have traced the outer edge of your bubble, or kinesphere, and you are standing within that bubble, with yourself at the center and with stars above you, below you, to the right side, to the left side, in front of you, and behind you. Now that you've outlined that space, stand in that space and feel it. Claim that wonderful personal space for yourself.

- Sweep your arms along the inner walls of your bubble, down, and then in front of you and behind you, feeling the edges of your space.

- From there, reach diagonally, continuing to trace the inner edges of your bubble up and down, first with your right hand and then with your left.

- Continue to fill in the rest of your bubble, stretching your arms and moving through each dimension, feeling every edge of your personal bubble, and enjoying that wonderful reach.

- Now close your eyes and imagine that that your whole personal bubble is filled with a mist. Take a moment to visualize the entire depth and breadth of the space within your bubble.

- Next, fill that mist with a beautiful primary color. Take note of what color you see in your mind's eye. Is it purple? Is it yellow? Is it orange? Imagine that you're like the Good Witch in *The Wizard of Oz*, floating down in your beautiful bubble, safely surrounded by the colored mist. As you do that, really claim that space. Take a moment to really enjoy it.

- Slowly open your eyes and adjust to your surroundings, appreciating how it feels to really experience your kinesphere and own the dynamic space all around you.

- You might also do this exercise facing a partner, with plenty of space between you, so that you can feel the edges of your personal bubbles against each other, feeling your energy bouncing off each other. You might

SEEING OURSELVES

even try and guess their color. Enjoy this feeling of understanding each other's space: claiming your own while experiencing the edge of theirs.

- You can then take a step forward and explore how it feels to have your bubbles overlap and share your kinespheres.

- Now you've experienced this beautiful space, let go of your bubble, letting the stars float back in toward you and gently dissolve into your heart.

- Take a deep breath and come back into the room, reflecting on how it felt to visualize your space.

- How does it feel to inhabit the space that you're in?

- Are you standing differently than you were at the start of the exercise?

- Take a moment to reflect on the experience of owning your kinesphere.

When you consciously own your space, it allows you to be more discerning about how to inhabit the space, how you interact with other people's space, and how you allow other people to enter your space. When working with actors, I invite them to try this exercise to explore conscious choices about how they place themselves in relationship with others. Entering someone's space can be confronting; we typically soften the lines between us and face each other at a diagonal rather than squarely head on to lessen that feeling of confrontation. For actors, sharing kinespheres in these different ways helps them understand the physicality of their interactions. As nonactors we can also apply this understanding to how we engage with each other.

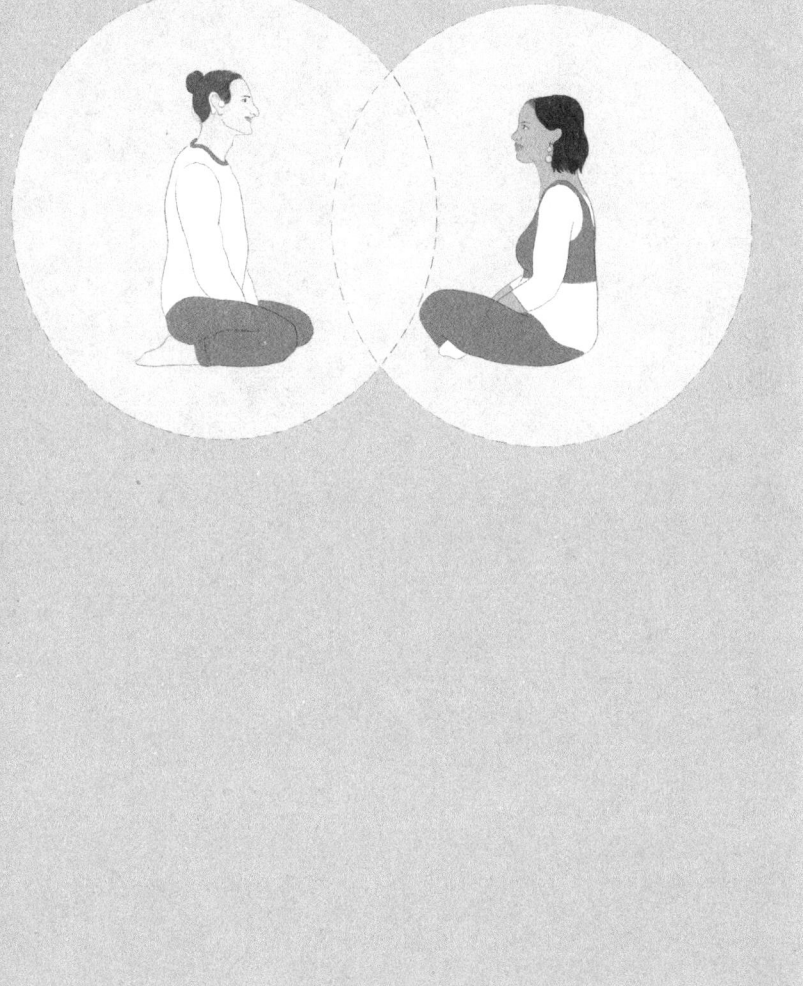

CHAPTER FIVE

CALLING OUR BOUNDARIES, GIVING CONSENT

There is a scene in Michaela Coel's *I May Destroy You* that—even though I had a hand in creating it—told me something I didn't know. Arabella has sex with a character called Zain, who appears to be likable and caring. They have explicitly agreed to have sex and Arabella has asked him to use a condom; during intercourse from behind, he pulls out and removes the condom, and then re-enters. They continue to have sex, but it has changed from protected sex to unprotected sex, without Arabella's knowledge and, therefore, without her consent.

When Arabella, a writer by profession, finds out that Zain has deliberately removed the protection, she reveals her anger at a literary conference. "He's not rape adjacent or a bit rapey, he's a rapist under UK law."

I was shocked because until I worked on *I May Destroy You*, I didn't realize that removing a condom without your partner's consent—known as stealthing—did actually count as rape in the UK and some other countries, including Germany. The scene is a particularly important example of the responsibility that art has toward being honest and truthful. By creating work that deals with different kinds of abuse, Coel is dramatizing and explaining what that abuse is.

The entire series of *I May Destroy You* had such an impact because it managed to tell its story with a sure grip on dealing with issues of sexual assault and abuse while simultaneously painting a vivid picture of a group of friends from the Black British community in London negotiating a world where such issues are an everyday occurrence.[1] It did all this with a lightness of touch and a seriousness of purpose that marked it out as something incredibly special.

As an article in the *Guardian* in July 2020 pointed out: "While sexual assault is not the focus of every interaction, or every scene, it does provide the backdrop from which everything else emerges. Its quiet presence shows sexual abuse as something that exists inside our world rather than a threat from somewhere far away—something you or I or anyone else may have experienced without even realizing it was happening."[2]

The series is immensely valuable because it reveals, in mainstream entertainment, how abuse and sexual assault happens. It makes it absolutely clear that as soon as someone becomes predatory and either takes away your ability to set boundaries and to say no or yes to a sexual encounter, or simply refuses to listen to your no, the encounter is no longer about intimacy, it is about power. It is not about loving and wanting connection, it is about one person inflicting their power over another.

This is incredibly important to state: intimate relationships involve consent. They do not involve one person overriding another person's wishes. There's no better guide to what consent means than the video, widely shared by the police in the UK but originally created by Blue Seat Studios and blogger Rockstar Dinosaur Pirate Princess, that asks people to imagine that instead of initiating sex, they are asking someone if they would like a cup of tea. If someone says yes, I would like a cup of tea, then you know they want a cup of tea. If they say they are not sure, you might make them a cup of tea—but you wouldn't force them to drink it. If they say no, then they just don't want tea.

Even if they initially say yes, but when the tea arrives, they've decided they don't want tea at all, you mustn't get annoyed. They remain under no obligation to drink the tea. It is OK for people to change their mind. You are not entitled to watch them drink it. If they are unconscious—as in Arabella's story—don't make them tea. Unconscious people don't want tea and they can't answer the question yes or no, because they weren't conscious when you asked.

Even if they said yes when they were conscious, if they are unconscious when you bring the tea, then check to make sure they are all right. And—this is the important part—don't make them drink the tea or keep pouring it down their throat. Unconscious people don't want tea. Equally, if someone said yes to tea at your house last Saturday, it doesn't necessarily mean they want tea all the time. You can't go to their house unexpectedly, make them tea, and force them to drink it.

If you can understand how completely ludicrous it is to force people to have tea when they don't want tea, and if you understand what they say when they say no to a cup of tea, then how difficult is it to understand a "no" when it comes to sex? Consent is everything. The tea scenarios I've just described from this brilliant little video entirely does away with the confusion people think arises when it comes to sexual assault.[3]

Equally, consent is explored in a short film on which I was the intimacy coordinator called *Keep Breathing*,[4] where a woman leaving her workplace at the end of the day gets trapped in a lift with a man who had invited himself into her flat at the end of their first date, and forced her to have sex. He won't take no for an answer and uses coercion tactics to override her resistance until she gives up and reluctantly endures sex.

He doesn't think he has done anything wrong; she knows that she said no, and that he continued to force himself on her anyway. She didn't fight back, feeling that it was better just to go through with sex than to risk violence. In the lift with him, the fictional protagonist finds the courage to say that she didn't want sex with him that night—that her no meant no. He is shocked. He sees himself as a good person, not a rapist. The implication is that he will consider his actions in future.

Keep Breathing is a wonderfully crafted and acted film about perception, miscommunication, and how one person can feel a date is going really well and yet the other person sees it from a very different viewpoint. Its aim—and its effect—is to promote discussion and understanding. If you watch it with friends, you might very well find that you can easily spend an hour or two discussing what you've just seen, and that you might not all agree on what it means.

Such confusion arises in a society where different forms

of harassment are the norm. A UN survey in 2023 revealed that 97 percent of 18- to 24-year-olds in the UK had experienced harassment in public places and more than 70 percent of women of all ages had endured such behavior. And of all men, one in six will have experienced some harassment or abuse.[5] According to statistics compiled by the job search organization Zippia, it's estimated that 54 percent of women have experienced some form of sexual harassment in the workplace, including behavior such as unwanted touching, requests for sexual favors, catcalls, and sexually suggestive gestures.[6]

For the LGBT community, according to a study by the Williams Institute at UCLA School of Law, "LGBT people are nearly four times more likely than non-LGBT people to experience violent victimization, including rape, sexual assault, and aggravated or simple assault."[7]

However, between 58 percent and 72 percent of victims do not report this because they are worried about retaliation, possible job loss, or being known as a troublemaker. Meanwhile, the US Equal Employment Opportunity Commission (EEOC) says that from 2018 to 2021, the total number of sexual harassment charges rose 3 percent over the previous three years, while a 2018 study by the nonprofit Stop Street Harassment found that 81 percent of women surveyed had been victims of sexual harassment.[8] That same study reported that 77 percent of women had experienced verbal sexual harassment, 51 percent had been sexually touched without permission, 41 percent said they had been sexually harassed online, and 27 percent said they had survived sexual assault. A survey from the Office for National Statistics in the UK further found that one in four women and one in six to seven men will be victims of domestic abuse in their lifetime.[9] As I said, and as I want to reiterate, these are not intimate encounters. They are about power, not about sex. A no is a no. A no means stop. But the difficulty of calling your boundaries, of insisting on what you want rather than going along with someone else's desires, persists both in intimate and abusive situations. Consent is directly related to being able to call your boundaries—and knowing what those boundaries are.

One of the essential parts of my work is conducting actor "check-ins" where I invite the actor to share their requirements for the intimate content of each scene. In a workshop session, to help an actor to become aware of where their boundaries are regarding touch, I often use an exercise where two people stand opposite each other and ask permission to touch different parts of the other person's body. There is no actual touch, just the request, with the partner really considering the question and then responding. For example, "Is it all right if I hold your right hand in my left?" "Is it OK if I put both my hands on your shoulders?" "Is it all right if I put my forehead on your shoulder?" "May we hug, chest to chest?" "May we hug, belly to belly?"

It is important to put parameters in place for this exercise, even though there is no actual touch, as an imagined action can be as profound as an actual experience of touch. There are no requests to put a body part into another person's body part, and breasts and the pelvic region/genital area are out of bounds.

The first time the questions are asked, you respond with a yes to every request, giving you an opportunity to listen to your internal physical reactions. When the requests are repeated, you respond with a no. At no point is there any physical contact. But in every instance, you have to consider whether you really want to go ahead with what the other person is asking. If I ask, for example, "Is it OK if I put my nose on your belly?" your automatic response may well be a no, but in this exercise, you are exploring what saying yes might feel like.

The exercise is a revelation because it gives you the opportunity for your inner body wisdom to let you understand what is and is not OK for you. It becomes absolutely clear when the word you are saying may be yes, yet every fiber of the body is communicating a no and vice versa. It is most revealing and enlightening, and at the same time, it can be very funny. If you learn to trust the body, it knows what is OK; it knows the yes and the no. The exercise, which I took from Betty Martin's *Wheel of Consent*,[10] enables you to call your boundaries in a deep and meaningful way.

All too often, in life and in making art, we say yes because it's easy, or because it seems polite, but really, we are screaming no inside. We're ignoring what our body is telling us. You can actually observe this in people's physical reactions. Once when I was giving a workshop in Stockholm, I was supporting the actors through the process of agreement and consent of touch. We were rehearsing a scene that contained a moment of intimate touch and a kiss. One actor asked another whether they could touch their acting partner's hair. She said yes, but as her partner gently stroked her hair, her body responded with a reaction, like a shiver, where every single cell was activated, and to her own intense surprise, she began to cry.

As I always do, I'd set a time-out system in place before

we began working, so she was able to call time-out and we took a break to allow her to process what had happened. The actor had no idea that someone touching her hair wouldn't be OK for her. As we began the work again, we established that the hair was a no but discovered that the request from her acting partner to touch her cheek—in many ways a more intimate gesture—was absolutely fine.

Everyone has different boundaries, and it is not our right to ask why they might be in place. I didn't need to know why that particular actor found having her hair touched so disturbing, just as I don't need to know why every actor has a different relationship with performing with a degree of nudity. The process of the guidelines allows a performer to call their boundaries with no questions asked. The principle of engaging with your nervous system and finding out what your body is telling you helps to set the rules with which we engage with other people. Try it with your partner or a friend. It is always a voyage of discovery.

This separation between mind and body emerges in different ways. After my father died, I told everyone that I was fine, and gave myself very little time to process the shock and sadness of his death. I talked about it quite freely and openly, without any particular problem. Yet when I started to describe the circumstances of his death to a friend, my voice began to crack and tears came. My body was telling me something my mind was ignoring.

One way or another, we very often override our own instinctive reactions. Before the implementation of the Intimacy on Set Guidelines, it might have been that in an audition, when asked, an actor would fear not taking their top off because they felt that if they didn't, they wouldn't be considered for a part. On a film set, someone might not have wanted to say no even when they didn't want to perform an intimate scene because they were worried that they would be seen as difficult and obstructive.

The actor Sofia Helin, star of television's *The Bridge*, remarked in a discussion about sets where no intimacy coordinator was present: "It's tense every time you have to cross your own borders in order to satisfy a director's needs . . . What we as actors want to do is to tell the story and we can do almost anything to tell the story, especially when the team is there and the camera is on. You say 'yes' to almost anything just to serve the story. So that 'no' has to be listened to by someone who can just step in and say 'No, no. We don't do that.' "[11]

As Helin's remarks show, part of the reason for the creation of the Intimacy on Set Guidelines was to give actors a professional way in which they could call their boundaries as part of the creative process. This is just the same as an actor saying I am afraid of heights if they are asked to jump off a roof and then having that respected and accommodated, either by employing a stunt performer, or by filming the scenes in any number of creative ways.

It's not only on a film set that boundaries are regularly breached. Similar problems arise in so many workplaces. A lot of women will recognize the moment when a male colleague places a hand on a shoulder or an arm—or even around a waist—when he is talking to you. It feels uncomfortable, but from a reluctance to make things awkward, or perhaps from a sense that if you say anything it will count against you, you just go along with it.

Or perhaps putting yourself in line for promotion for a new job involves joining in activities that make you feel unhappy. Perhaps as a nondrinker, you feel compelled to go to the wine bar with your colleagues and be on the sidelines while they get drunk, when if you had actually been asked what you wanted to do, you'd have gone home and watched TV. Even worse, maybe you come under attack because you won't drink, and feel pressured to breach your personal choices in order to be a part of the workplace culture. All too often it is the person who says "that is inappropriate" rather than the one who just goes along with the flow, against all their better judgment, who is seen as being prudish or touchy or unprofessional, when in fact it is the person applying the pressure who is in the wrong.

In an ideal world, the call would be for all workplaces to implement systems for dealing with such microaggressions; for all offices to set up independent and effective human resources departments and procedures that protect the rights of all their employees; and for employees to be able to call out inappropriate behavior without fear of repercussions and be supported throughout the process.

A positive work environment encourages all employees to call their boundaries in order to create working systems that benefit and protect everyone. A code of conduct, openly communicated, and a path to address breaches in the code, which means that everyone knows that they will be treated with respect and in confidence when they bring up a problem, is in fact a recipe for professional and happier working.

There are some good guidelines that can be followed in a working environment that avoid abusive patterns and protect the areas of risk. For example, it is never appropriate for someone in a junior role to be asked by someone in a senior role to work outside hours in their private home. It is never appropriate to sexually objectify anyone's body, whether that's in a rehearsal room or an office, or for any colleague to be made to feel exposed by comments on their appearance in any way.

It is inappropriate in any setting to send overly personal or suggestive communications, particularly to a junior colleague, but also to a peer, unless it is quite clear that comments of this sort are wanted. It's inappropriate to initiate unwanted intimate physical contact—and people should be careful about physical contact of any kind in a work situation, especially from a senior to a more junior colleague. Only hug people who you really know well and who clearly want to be hugged, putting in place a gesture or verbal request and waiting for a positive response before acting on the offer. In the same way, it is rarely appropriate in a general work setting to ask people about their personal experiences; if they offer them, that is one thing, but don't expect them to share. It is about respecting the personal self and the professional self. A person's personal self is just that, personal, and to be respected as private.

These are broad codes of behavior, but they are relatively simple to bear in mind and they make workplaces safer and more professional.

It is all about knowing that our boundaries are to be respected and to become practiced in listening to and calling our boundaries. It's not so much a question of leaning in as it is of standing your ground, asserting your right to be heard, making sure that what your body is telling you about what you need is communicated to those around you. As I've said, the first step is to be present in your body, to listen to its impulses and responses, and then find a way of outlining what they are.

However, this takes practice in feeling confident to speak up. For a long period of my life, I felt I struggled with this. When I trained as an actor at the Bristol Old Vic, I had difficulties with sight-reading. When I first read a script, it felt as if it was scrambled. (Only many years later was I diagnosed as dyslexic.) Added to this, my teachers thought the tone of my voice sounded as if I might be partially deaf. I was told about the work of Alfred Tomatis and chose to embark on a two-week course following the alternative medicine theories of hearing and listening known as Audio-Psycho-Phonology (APP).[12]

This is a listening program that develops motor, emotional, and cognitive skills by stimulating the inner ear in order to restore listening. The idea is that if the communication between the ear and the brain is blurred, our ability to interact with the outside world is compromised. But it can be improved. Just as you can reengage your stomach muscles by doing exercises, so can you reengage the inner ear through the methods Tomatis developed. For two weeks, I was put on an intensive program of listening to filtered Gregorian chanting and to Mozart. There is some skepticism about this method, but for me it was incredible. I felt it had a huge impact in waking up my ear—and so improving the resonance of my voice. It seemed to awaken things. Because I felt more confident, I could trust that my voice could communicate the emotions I wanted to convey as I took on different acting roles. I had more control over how I was speaking.

It's incredibly important for us not only to have confidence in our bodies (as I've explained earlier) but also to find a voice, not just metaphorically but physically. In my exploration of work, in the rehearsal process I often use sounding as part of the warm-up, engaging in practices such as chakra toning and overtone chanting. For this, we return to the energy centers that I outlined in Chapter Three.

I first experienced this practice when I attended a week-long workshop with Jill Purce, who works with ancient Mongolian overtone chanting. (See further information on the workshop and the technique on page 159.) It's a wonderful practice to do every day. "Overtone chanting has been used as a healing tool in some ancient religions," according to Purce, who says that the overtones have a power that operates all the way from consciousness down to the cellular level.[13] Vowels carry the information energy of speech, whereas consonants act to break the energy flow. They carry the intention and force of what we are saying. I tend to ask participants to work in pairs to do the exercises, but you can quite easily do them alone, sitting comfortably in a chair or on a cushion on the floor, with your spine as straight as possible so that energy flows through your body more easily. The suggestion is to sound into each chakra for seven breaths, through the sounds *uuh, ooo, oh, ah, eh, aye, eee*. Explore with the sound as gently as possible, so as not to strain, and to find the correct pitch for each particular chakra, scanning up and down, feeling in your body for the resonance.

I used this exercise when I was in rehearsals working on *Does My Sex Offend You?*, a theater piece that explored the relationship between perpetrators and their victims. Very often, in experiences of abuse a person is devoiced, so I wanted to discover ways of reclaiming the voice. After we had sounded through the energy centers connecting with the different vowel sounds, we repeated the same exercise but replaced the vowel sounds with "No." I wanted to explore how the different energy centers affected the quality of the "No." Giving about two to three minutes to explore each sound, we played with the quality, emotion, and physicality of the "No," and then came to stillness, feeling the resonance of the experience in each center. We anchored the discoveries in drawing an image on paper of the quality of each exploration.

We discovered that a no that came from the base of the spine was incredibly raw and fierce, for example; the real sound of the survival instinct, an absolute rejection. The sound of the "No" when it came from the second sacral chakra, our emotional center, sounds like women wailing in grief. The solar plexus is responsible for confidence and self-esteem, as well as helping you to feel in control of your life. The emotions associated with this energy center are excitement, happiness, depression, and anger. The "No" from this center has a sense of standing up for yourself and declaring who you are in the world.

When the "No" came from the heart, it could be gentle and loving as well as firm, like the no a parent would say to stop a child from putting their hands in the fire. When the "No" came from the throat, it expressed a clear presence by communicating what you want. From the brow, the "No" took on a different, more intellectual quality, and by the time the "No" reached the top of the head, it had an almost spiritual tone.

Exploring where the "No" sits in our body and giving voice to it is incredibly powerful—and extraordinarily empowering. After one workshop, a participant, Sue Appleby, wrote thanking me for a positive and vulnerable experience. "When talking with my [workshop] partner about a strong no I had given, I wrote down the following feelings that accompanied it: conviction, purity, power/strength, vulnerability/fear, honesty, clarity, liberation."

The workshop, she said, had taught her the importance of following her instinct and knowing when to say no. "I just need to believe that my needs and desires are important, just as important as those around me. I've been trying this out over the past day or so and it feels good. As well as leading to greater authenticity, less suffering or martyrdom, it is generally happy making!"[14]

Learning to say no and calling your boundaries can be truly liberating and lead to a happier existence both in intimate relationships and work settings. In another workshop, after completing the "No" exercise, a different participant said that they went home and turned down a job they had been thinking of accepting because they felt they ought to. They knew, in their gut, that it was the wrong position for them, and yet had hesitated because it seemed wrong to refuse work. Another person said that the exercise had helped them say "No" when a friend asked them to go out, when they really wanted to stay in.

Like any muscle, it takes practice to exercise your "No," have it in your mouth, get ready to discover its different qualities. Saying no gently, for example, doesn't have to be a negative thing. It can be positive and loving. It helps other people to know you and understand who you are and what you want.

The other thing I should stress about this calling of boundaries is that being clear about your "No," being able to state your "No," means that your "Yes" can be trusted. If you are invited to state your requirements, and give your consent to what you are doing, then when you say yes, people know that the affirmative is truly and freely given. Your "No" is a gift, because it means we can trust your "Yes" and can be confident that you are taking responsibility for yourself.

That's the entire point about open communication and agreement and consent as a starting point for the Intimacy on Set Guidelines in the entertainment industry. It is so true in our lives too. If we set a frame for our behavior, then it enables us to communicate honestly and truthfully. In relationships, we're often trying to make a good impression—especially in our early encounters.

The simplest example I can think of is the person who pretends they love soccer because they want to be with someone who is obsessed with sports. It seems such a simple remark, but if the relationship develops, then strains can develop because of the pretense. They may find all their spare time is devoted to following Arsenal or Manchester United—and because they haven't called their boundaries, then problems arise.

If your intention is to have a lovely, intimate time with someone, then the way you are going to have a nicer time is by encouraging open communication from the very start. Misunderstandings are so easy, especially if you don't explain things. Once again, the screen can provide us with instances of how to be honest and open with people and how to engage in difficult conversations before confusion arises.

I am thinking of examples such as the scene in the series *Sex Education,* in season two, where two male gay characters are about to have sex for the first time. The more experienced of the two refuses to have anal sex until the other has sorted out his anal hygiene. He calls his boundaries, says what he wants—and the result is that the other character goes away, finds out about what he needs to do, and they then have a successful sexual encounter.

In *Euphoria* (which I didn't work on), a teenage couple are having sex for the first time, and the boy suddenly starts behaving in a way that is completely out of character—being dominant and aggressive because that is how he has seen men behave in the pornography he has watched. When the girl tells him to stop, he is confused. He thinks he is doing the right thing. Her "No" helps him to understand what she really wants from an intimate relationship.

None of this is easy. It can be hard to define what you want. But if in our relationships we put the invitation in place, then it is easier to communicate with each other and discover deeper intimacy—which is based on consent. This doesn't prevent people exploring new experiences or embarking on different journeys. It is difficult to suggest something new or groundbreaking in an intimate relationship when you are actually in the throes of sex, although it is always better to say something rather than staying silent. It's much better, however, to find a way to express what you might want to explore and ask your partner what they are into beforehand. Then check in with your sexual partner afterward, asking whether there was anything they would like to have happened differently. Intimate relationships can keep developing in life when couples have found a way to be truthful with each other, so that they understand each other's needs.

I invite you to practice talking and expressing yourself in this way, so it becomes part of your relationship and deepens your intimacy. Another invitation is to give yourselves the gift of time, to create an atmosphere of openness. I think in most people's rushed lives, they don't always create the space simply to be with each other, without expectation. Every encounter doesn't have to end in sex. Sometimes it can simply be about having a meal or giving each other a massage. The important thing is that you are aware of each other.

This brings me back to Betty Martin and the Wheel of Consent. When the actor in Stockholm shivered when her acting partner touched her hair, it wasn't my place in that professional setting to find out why the gesture was activating for her. In a workplace, it is not required to know the story behind someone's instinctive reaction. In life, and in relationships, it often really helps develop further intimacy if you do.

Betty Martin, who is a sexologist and intimacy coach, has used the wheel to guide clients in their relationships; she now offers mentoring for a wide range of practitioners who use touch. In the development of her ideas—which she generously makes available online to anybody who wants to study them—she divides touch into four quadrants, distinguishing between who is doing the touch and who it's for. You can touch your partner the way they want, or the way you want, and the difference is significant. On the other side, your partner can touch you the way they want or the way you want—also a significant difference. She says all four are wanted and needed, as long as there is agreement.[15]

If you move this into practical examples, then if I am upset, and I need a hug, I am eliciting touch because I need it. If I come home and I notice my partner is stressed, then I am giving touch for them.

As you think through the examples on the wheel, you begin to understand the difference between giving and

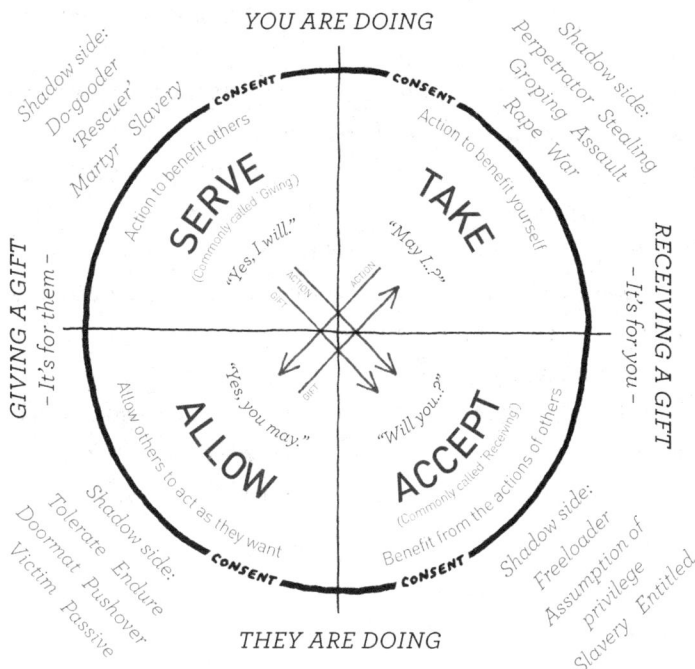

receiving touch and hold that awareness in yourself. That feels like a revelation in terms of understanding the quality of touch.

Even when I facilitate agreement and consent of touch in warm-ups and workshops, I notice subtle differences in how people react to each other. People will respond differently to the questions depending on who is asking them—they might be happy to give a body hug to one person but not to another. Two women working through the exercise might reveal different sensations than a woman and a man, or two men. In terms of my work, that is important to know. It means that when I am choreographing scenes for individuals, I can respect their boundaries. They can feel supported in giving a yes with one person, and a no with another.

In life, of course, this often goes to the root of human attraction. We want to be with some people and not with others. We might react not only to their bodies but to the pheromones they give off, that hidden form of communication that triggers different hormonal reactions and conditions how we react to each other. Exploring touch and hormonal reactions in this way is an important part of is an important part of intimacy.

It does, however, very much come back to living in our own bodies and responding to what they tell us, which is part of what interests me and which will be the subject of the next chapter.

TONING THROUGH THE ENERGY CENTERS OF THE BODY

I first experienced sounding through the body and overtone chanting at a week-long workshop that I attended run by Jill Purce in April 1995. I have since used these sounding techniques with my actors as part of the warm-up before embarking on rehearsals. I also took the basis of this practice and used it to explore the power of "No" with my students and actors.

This exercise supports you in finding connection, empowerment, and self-knowing through resonating and balancing the energy centers located along the midline of the body, or chakras, using vowel sounds, and then to explore the "No" from each of these places in the body to understand how you can connect with your vulnerability and state your boundaries through the "No."

- To practice chakra toning, start by sitting comfortably in a chair or on a cushion on the floor that supports you to keep your spine as straight as possible, which allows the energy to flow more freely through the body.

- When engaging with the toning, you can either close your eyes or hold a soft gaze to focus on the sensation.

- Explore the sounding in each energy center through seven breaths. Focus the first four breaths to find your connection with the energy center through the vowel sounds, and the next three to explore saying and sounding "No" in that pitch.

- Allow yourself to investigate the pitch in each energy center, allowing your voice to follow what feels most suitable for each chakra. Make these sounds in a gentle voice without straining your vocal cords.

- As you work through the body, it may also help to bring the hands to the relevant position in the body. If you are inspired to move, allow yourself to follow the physical impulses.

- Breathe in deeply, expanding your lower stomach as you inhale. Imagine the energy of each breath coming into your body through whichever chakra you are working on; this may help you to focus your awareness.

- As you are toning, allow yourself to focus on the sound, and if you find your mind has wandered, that's fine; just bring your focus back again to the sound you are making.

- As you complete the sounding in each chakra, allow yourself to come to silence and stillness, experiencing what resonates through you, and bring your awareness to any thoughts or feelings that may have come up, before moving onto the next chakra.

- **First chakra (Base):** located at the base of the spine. Tone four times with the deepest "UUH," as in "pull"; it will feel like a very low guttural sound just gently riding on the breath. Stay comfortable with the sound—don't force it. Then find your "No" in this register three times.

- **Second chakra (Sacral):** located about 2–3 inches below the navel. Tone four times using a slightly higher pitch but still being a deep "OOO," as in "you." Then find your "No" in this register three times.

- **Third chakra (Solar plexus):** located above the navel, just below the ribs. Tone four times using a higher pitched "OH," as in "go." Then find your "No" in this register three times.

- **Fourth chakra (Heart):** located in the center of the chest. Tone four times using a higher pitched "AH," as in "ma." This is the sound that embodies compassion. Then find your "No" in this register three times.

- **Fifth chakra (Throat):** located in the throat. Tone four times using a higher pitched "EH," as in "egg." Then find your "No" in this register three times.

- **Sixth chakra (Third eye):** located in the middle of the forehead, slightly above the eyes. Tone four times using a still higher "AYE," as in "eye." Then find your "No" in this register three times.

- **Seventh chakra (Crown):** located at the top of the skull. Tone four times using the highest pitched "EEE" sound, as in "me," you can comfortably make. Then find your "No" in this register three times.

- Once you have completed the toning and exploring with your "No" through all seven chakras, allow

CALLING OUR BOUNDARIES, GIVING CONSENT

yourself to come to silence and stillness, experiencing what resonates through you.

- What images, thoughts, and sensations did you encounter?

- How did you feel during the exercise?

- Did any memories come to you?

- When you feel you have given yourself enough time to reflect on the exercise, open your eyes if they are not already open, bring yourself back into the space, and enjoy stretching through your body.

- If it works for you, a good way to anchor your experience is to write any thoughts or reflections in a notebook or to draw any images, shapes, and colors that came to you.

CHAPTER SIX

THE SENSUOUS BODY

In January 2023, I was invited to be part of a panel discussion at the Sundance Film Festival chaired by the psychoanalyst Dr. Orna Guralnik, who hosts the hugely popular TV series *Couples Therapy*. Her show closely follows four couples over six months of weekly treatment, giving viewers a deep insight into the experience of couples therapy. During the panel discussion, Guralnik's opening gambit was to ask us how we defined intimacy in our lives, and my fellow panelist, the film director Barry Jenkins, said something really interesting.

He said that in his personal relationships, he was trying to strip away the performative aspects of intimacy. "I know what I want to be saying and what I should be saying in here right now, but I also know what I am feeling . . . I am trying to de-intellectualize it . . . and just be intimate without performing it," he said. "It is communication and getting to the state of being where you are just present. Maybe intimacy . . . is just pure, honest presence."[1]

Yet achieving that state of presence is one of the hardest things to do. Our entire lives are often based on being in two places at once: checking our phone messages while we are talking to someone or picking the kids up from school while ordering the groceries online or chatting to a friend on the telephone while at the same time reading the headlines. We pride ourselves on our ability to multitask, to push on with many activities at the same moment.

At the same time, contemporary existence is pushing us further and further from our own bodies, creating a disassociation between what we are feeling and what we are doing. We can be sitting by our computers, looking at travel photographs, or watching a film by moving nothing more than our fingertips. Instead of going outside to climb trees and roll around in the mud, turning sticks into weapons, our children can sit in a darkened room, with no fresh air, and wipe out entire battalions with a twitch of their thumbs.

In 2024, I was working on a stage adaptation of Frances Hodgson Burnett's 1911 novel, *The Secret Garden,* and as I reread the novel, I was bowled over by how far-sighted it is. It is a lot of people's favorite childhood book, and that's perhaps because it takes two children who are unloved and unlovable and leads them on a healing journey. In bringing an overgrown garden back to life, Mary and Colin return to nature, breathing in the air, having their hands in the soil, and being rejuvenated by the magic of the garden springing to life.

If that was true in 1911, how much truer it is today when modern technology holds us in our homes and disconnects us from experiencing life out in nature. It also separates us from our bodies. If you are busy recording on Instagram or TikTok the way something tastes and feels, you aren't giving yourself enough time to actually experience it. To live in the moment. To look at the sky. To listen to the bird song and feel the air on your skin. To taste the food instead of photographing it or describing it. Many people are so busy mediating their lives for public consumption that they have forgotten how to live them.

In *The Secret Garden,* the children's immersion in nature, in the moment-to-moment appreciation of the natural world—making space, clearing the weeds so that the plants have room to grow in the sunlight, the snowdrops pushing through, the robin in the tree—gives them a joy, wonder, and appreciation and love of life that makes them feel alive and therefore lovable. The same applies to intimacy. It is giving yourself time and space to be in your body. Being in your sensations, appreciating everything, allows you to be sensuous. If you close your eyes and simply listen for a few minutes, you can bring yourself back into your body and feel present. Or you could concentrate on what you can smell, or what you can feel, touching your clothes, your skin, your face. You could think about what you can taste in your mouth: Can you taste the air in some way? What can you hear? Can you hear the sound of the birds, the rush of the traffic, the breeze in the trees? Perhaps you deliberately look around you and note what you can see: the colors, the shapes. All these simple techniques help in encouraging a kind of mindfulness, pulling you back into the moment.

The same applies when you are with another person. Being in your body allows you to be aware of the sound of their breath, the rhythm of their breath, their smell. It allows you to connect with your gaze, both in terms of what you notice about them and their eye-to-eye connection. You can think about how they feel or that first touch of a hand.

Being in your body means you notice and respond to both your feelings and impulses and those of the person you are with, as the possibility of the desire to lean forward and kiss rises in you and in them. And in that kiss, what is the sensation as the lips meet for the first time? What is the texture and the taste? How is your desire communicating to them, and what are you receiving of their desire for you? This all springs from being grounded, of literally rooting ourselves and allowing different sensations to flow through our bodies, of bringing ourselves back to our basic primeval connection with the earth. One simple, mindful way of bringing this about, and an exercise I often use at the start of working with students, is to ask them to think of themselves as a tree. Everything from the waist downward is like the base of a tree, putting its roots down deep into the earth.

From the waist up, you are the branches of that tree, raising your arms, your head, your ribs, your chest up and out to the sun. Imagine yourself as a tall, beautiful column connecting earth and sky. Feel energy rising from the ground, flowing up through your spine and out the crown of your head. At the same time, sense the sun's energy entering through the crown, moving down your spine, and out through your feet, extending like deep roots into the earth's core.

That image and feeling of groundedness is incredibly important for helping us be present. Once you are rooted to the earth in this way, then your breath starts to flow more freely through your body. It is important in intimate relations because it places you in the moment when you interact with another person, either partner or friend, totally aware of them in the space around you.

A fun way to experience the positive effects of being

grounded with a friend or partner is to have a go at the "Seaweed Exercise." Working in pairs, one of you imagines that you're seaweed floating in the sea, and the other a little fish. If you are the seaweed, imagine you're in the sea, allowing the currents of the water to move you gently, and then a fish comes along and just nudges you; allow yourself to go with the movement, relaxing your body, feeling where that nudge takes you. The fish can push you in your knees, or hips, or shoulders, or a hand, and if you're the seaweed, imagine how you will move and also be carried by the water around you so you come floating back.

After a little while, the fish swims away and the seaweed carries on imagining what it feels like to be floating and what it was like to be nudged by the fish.

Now, imagine yourself as seaweed anchored into the seabed, sending its roots down through the sand, and going down, down, down into the seabed, wrapping around boulders, which pull you down and anchor you so you have a solid connection with the ocean floor but can still undulate in the water. The fish comes along again and nudges you, in your elbows, or on your head, or in your back, or in your knees. This time, feel how you are moved by the fish but your roots are deep down. How does this feel when you are moved but anchored and secure?

Then the fish swims away! Close your eyes and allow yourself to feel what it was like to feel this with roots that allowed you to be firm into the ground. Then open your eyes and swap over.

Exercises such as this are a way of expanding sensory experience and through the play understand the qualities that groundedness gives you and how you can take this understanding and experience into your daily life. For example, when you are meeting with your partner at a restaurant for a "date night," but your mind is still full of the concerns from your day at work, and you are not able to give your full attention to your lover. Take the time to let go of where you have been, perhaps even using the technique of running water on your wrists that we spoke about in an earlier chapter, grounding yourself by sending your roots down as in the fish exercise, and then set your intention on the time you have created to nurture your relationship. This will allow you to walk into the restaurant, letting your partner know that you only have eyes for them, and that you are there, body, mind, and soul, to enjoy a loving time together.

In contemplating the experience of being grounded, sending roots from your feet into the earth, the shoes that you wear can make a huge difference to how you can connect to the earth through your feet.

The pressures and expectations of society and Hollywood for how to look and what to wear, as we have spoken about in an earlier chapter, can also have a strong influence on our sense of presence.

As Florence Pugh remarked in December 2024, "It's really exhausting for a young woman to just be in this industry . . . There are fine lines women have to stay within . . . it's always been fashionable to tell a woman how she should live her life."[2]

One of my concerns with the entire red-carpet syndrome, with the way women are encouraged to present themselves in the world, is that they so often are pressured to wear high heels. At the Cannes Film Festival, this reluctance to allow women to wear flats (the festival organizers claim they can wear any shoe as long as it is "smart") has prompted a pushback from participants such as Kristen Stewart, who, in 2016, very deliberately took off her spiky-heeled Louboutins as she walked up the red carpet. I notice that more women, on the red carpet and off, are choosing to wear flat shoes and sneakers.

It's an encouraging trend because, in my opinion, high heels are one of the principal barriers that stop women from feeling grounded. They are literally designed to accentuate certain properties in the body: the curve of the breasts and the buttocks.

According to Enrico Cuini, a shoe designer, "High heels adjust lumbar curvature, or the posture of your spine, increase pelvic tilt, and enhance the appearance of the chest and hips, all of which contribute to men perceiving a woman's gait in heels as more erotic and beautiful."[3]

High heels also accentuate that sense of women somehow being delicate, falling beings, taken away from their own sense of self by their footwear. That stereotype is repeated onscreen where women are always falling over their own feet. Look at Sarah Jessica Parker's character Carrie in the early incarnations of Sex and the City, a hugely influential series for so many women. She literally trips around New York, constantly falling, in a state of instability and flux.

Of course, if people want to wear heels, that is their choice. But it would be great if there was more awareness of the image they project and why. Our feet are important to our sense of who we are, yet we often ignore them and treat the incredible mechanism of bone, tendon, and muscle as if it is indestructible. Wearing high heels asks them to function in an unnatural manner, pushing the entire weight of the body down through the big toe joint, stretching the arch of the foot and distorting its shape in a way that is not so dissimilar from the old practice of foot binding.

After I had completed my MA in Movement Studies (2006–7) in 2010, I co-authored a paper called "From Grounded Foot to Leaping Foot" with Debbie Green, who was then a senior lecturer in movement for actors at the Royal Central School of Speech and Drama.[4]

The research looked at the training of the feet for actors, from being grounded, through to the training and articulation needed to allow them to jump and leap, and back to landing again. As our starting point, we took a quotation from the theater director Tadashi Suzuki, whose training method emphasizes what he calls "the grammar of the feet." He says: "A performance begins when the actor's feet touch the ground . . . when he first had the sensation of putting down roots; it begins in another sense when he lifts himself lightly from the spot."[5]

A lot of the exercises we collated were strongly technical, developed to help actors move from a grounded position to a jump and then back to earth again in safe and understandable ways. But one aspect of the study has a wider relevance to our intimate lives. The impulse of the leap is a basic human response, and we feel it in our intimate lives too, in the mind-body connection, where the stimulus, for instance, of seeing someone you love fills the body with a rising excitement and adrenaline as the sensation journeys up the spine.

The starting point to feeling this elation at its fullest, however, is to begin from a grounded position, an appreciation of your feet touching the earth. It's from there that the impetus to move up derives. It's important therefore not to ignore our feet but to lavish them with care and to understand how they work, as set out in the exercises at the end of Chapter Three. I've included an exercise at the end of this chapter to explore the articulation of the feet that will help you to understand the way movement travels from the feet through the body, helping you to make a leap of faith beyond the familiar.

When I am working with actors, once they have established a sense of groundedness, I ask them to imagine the actuality of their body, the structure of their bones, the feel of their muscle and their skin, the way that everything is connected. In order to encourage them to feel present in their bodies, I will build on the body awareness that I have described in previous chapters by using an exercise where we explore the elements—earth, fire, water, and air—that make up the world around us, and within us.

We start by exploring the element of the earth in our bodies; we feel into the bony structure of our skeleton, the cells that make up our organs, muscles, and skin. The consciousness of being in your body enhances the sense of touch; it enables you to relish and delight in the presence of another body next to you and how they feel. Then there is the sun, which is fire and energy, the nervous system that controls complicated processes like movement, thought, and memory, and regulates all the functions your body carries out without consciously thinking, like breathing and blinking. It also controls the impulses, which take on different qualities at different moments. If you think of impulses in terms of fire, when the fire is ignited, it's just the flicker of a candle flame, but then gradually it might grow into a bonfire, rising and rising, until it erupts like a volcano. If we are thinking about the way that the body moves to orgasm, then that sense of building in energy is a wonderful image.

Then there's air, which in our bodies is the breath of life, both aerobic and anaerobic. When we are talking about someone we have a crush on, or someone we admire, we often talk about them taking our breath away. When I talk about air in connection with the elements, I will often describe the way breath builds and also the way it sounds. If you are building a scene of intimacy, then that sounding, that sense of breath rising and falling, building to a climax, is the accompaniment to the recreation of sexual passion. In our own lives, if we listen to our own breathing and that of our intimate partners, we can tell what they are feeling.

It's the same with water, which is similar to air, but which has weight and momentum and which, in terms of the body, is all the fluid systems, the movement of the lymphatic and blood systems, moving oxygen, regulating the metabolism. Our bodily fluids include saliva, semen, vaginal fluids—all a natural part of intimacy. The initial connection with someone might feel like the trickle of a stream, but it later opens out into a river, then into a lake. Sometimes the lake is still, full of dark depths that you might imagine yourself diving into and exploring. Sometimes it is whipped up into waves, rising into a tsunami that crashes over us, leaving us spent. The parallel with orgasm is once again explicit.

Thinking of the elements, understanding them in our bodies, helps us feel ourselves as elemental beings. We are essentially animals of the earth, inextricably connected with the rhythm of the cycles, from day to night, the pull of the tides with the moon, the cycles of the seasons from winter, spring, summer, to autumn. That elemental sense of connection with the natural world is part of our fundamental human nature and our physicality.

As a starting point for this awareness, you can simply imagine the elements flowing through you and your reactions. When I am working with actors, I often suggest that they connect with the elements in the world around them. This was an exercise I was first introduced to in a workshop by Persis Jadé Maravala in 2008 and have since integrated into my practice.[6]

When I am building the intimate content with two actors, I will take them to a place in nature. Working as a pair, one of the participants closes their eyes, while the other gently guides them through the world around them. We live in nature all our lives, even if we live in cities of glass and steel. One place I used this exercise was with students in Hong Kong, and everyone thought I wouldn't be able to find any elements from the natural world in a city that was so built up. But you can. You always can. It's just that in our regular lives, we walk through nature without noticing it rather than appreciating it.

In Hong Kong, we found a beautiful area in between the high-rise blocks with patches of grass, water features, and bamboo sculptures. There I asked them to feel the different textures of the ground beneath their feet (this is particularly good if it is safe enough to take off your shoes), the change from the smooth floors of the studio to the hard ridges of the pavements.

Asking them to move in silence so that they are really present, I suggest they note the quality of the air, the transition from the stuffiness inside to the breeze on their faces as they step into the street.

When there isn't water available, we bring it in bottles with us so the actors can run the water on their hands, feel the different sensations of its flow, listening to the sounds of the waterdrops. I suggest that people plunge their hands into the earth, even if it's just a plant pot, feeling the soil, crushing a leaf from the plants growing to smell their aroma. Or they can feel a tree, the rough bark, the leaves on the branches. It is all about making a visceral connection with the world around us; after one of the pair has experienced it, they then swap over, guiding their partner through the elemental experience.

When both have completed the exercise, they walk back from the place in nature to the studio, walking in silence to keep the awareness of the sensations of the ground under their feet, the impact of the architecture around them, the noise of the cars if they have to cross a road, the shift in light when they walk back inside, the quality and smell of the air as they return.

There is nothing to pretend. You're just being present with the sensations, putting yourself in contact with nature and experiencing your own presence within it. Afterward, back in the studio, playing music, I invite the actors to close their eyes again and remember the experience, moving through from earth to fire, to water and air, connecting with the most vivid moments. Was it when they hugged a tree, or when they lay on the ground? Was it touching a flower? The warmth of the sun on their face, or the feeling of the gentle breeze over their arms? As you immerse yourself in the sensations, it completely alters your sense of where you are and how you feel.

I will ask people to dance these sensations, starting with the element of the earth, remembering the sensations of the ground, hands in the earth, the structure of the trees, the rise of the branches; then bringing that into the body, feeling the structure of their bones as they pushed themselves up from the floor. Moving on to the element of fire, and the connection with the sun, the feeling of light and shade on their skin, the heat in the body and the impulses of the nervous system, the electrical energy running through their body. Moving on to the element of water, feeling its trickle on their hands, or feet splashing in a puddle, the element of water mixing with the element of earth making mud; then connecting with the element of water in the body, with the momentum of the heartbeat and the flow of blood from the heart out to every cell in the body and back again into the heart. And, finally, the element of the air, connecting with the air on their skin, a breeze moving their clothes, and then connecting with the breath in the body, the rhythm of the breath, the air outside them being brought into them through the breath, and then breathing out contributing to the air around them.

With the actors in Hong Kong, one girl I taught said it made her realize how oppressed she felt by the traffic in the city, which she had never been aware of before; another noticed how she opened up when the sun hit her face.

The sense of presence that you can develop through an exercise like this is part of the preparation for intimacy. To some extent, we all make these accommodations subconsciously. If you are with someone you love, or with someone with whom you hope to establish intimacy, quite often you will soften the space around you, with candles or cushions or gentle lights. Not many people find it easy to be intimate in an environment of sharp, shiny surfaces. To relax, you want to create an atmosphere that feels womb-like, or cave-like, an environment that has a sense of warmth where you can soften, release, and let go. That's partly why in the buildup to the release of an orgasm, so many people close their eyes. They are looking inward, finding their inner connection in a journey toward release and sexual fulfillment.

But even at the stage of first meeting, the sensual perception of the elements is part of the intimacy. When you hold hands with someone, you're linking yourself to their nervous system and through that to the earth, which holds you both. Quite often you will go on a walk, immersing yourselves in nature, or go out for a meal, which again conjures the earthiness, the sheer, visceral pleasure of eating together, perhaps with a candle on the table, softening the atmosphere around you.

It is all part of the courting dance, a way of getting grounded together, of experiencing life. It is quite often, literally and metaphorically, a way of finding a shared space to be. In those early moments of going on dates, of establishing a relationship together, you are trying to work out whether the other person is the right one for you to spend intimate time with—and perhaps commit to for an ongoing relationship. You will want to know simple things: if you are at a point in your life where you want a baby, and the person you've just met doesn't, then you are not resonating in the same space. Those encounters are a means of gradually working out how you are both going to be within the same resonance, physically and emotionally.

But that sense of lived presence can be valuable in other ways too. When I was working on *Empire of Light*, there was a scene where a couple, waiting in line for cinema tickets, were kissing to the obvious discomfort of the cinema manager, played by Olivia Colman. All it said in the script was "they kiss," but it is difficult for actors just to be told to do that. It doesn't give them much sense of character within the scene and can be very uncomfortable.

To help them through, I broke the scene down into beats, describing who was kissing who at each point and with what intent. The choreography went something like this: she wants to be kissed so she kisses him, then breaks away; he pulls her back, and then they kiss again, exploring the touch of lips and the taste, then exploring the touch of bodies as the kiss deepens; and then they break.

A kiss is never just a kiss. It always holds something more within it. *My Lady Jane,* a TV drama series about the life of Lady Jane Grey on which I worked, was very much a kissing show, using the contact of a kiss to create complicated stories. For example, there was one scene where a couple were desperate to be together, and the woman hands the man a note expressing her feelings. He's overwhelmed and runs away, leaving her thinking she has done something awful. When she meets him again, sometime later, she lunges at him to make up, and he pulls back. But then he steps forward and kisses her with incredible passion; she kisses him back, and then they kiss long and hard. It is a lovely development of character, and it is entirely convincing as a series of kisses.

Obviously, in life, you're not going to count the length of time you kiss for, but part of being present is to be conscious of the significance and the feeling of that intimate contact. It's good rather than simply kissing to focus on the taste of another person, what their lips feel like, how they are communicating through their lips. It is like eating a peach; you want to feel and notice every moment.

Kissing is particularly important to women, I think, as a means of building connection and arousal. As the kissing becomes more passionate, endorphins are released that increase arousal. Anatomically, women don't get deeply aroused as quickly as men. They move from a phase of excitement in gradual stages until they are ready for full sexual engagement. I'm going to talk about this in more detail in a later chapter.

When I am choreographing an intimate scene onscreen, I try to build into the action an increasing intensity of heat, so that you see the stages of a sexual encounter rather than it looking like an instant reaction. In this context, kissing becomes more and more connected, through the lips and then exposing more skin, and then caressing other parts of the body. If you imagine it as a dance, it moves from the lips to the neck perhaps, to the taking off of clothes and to more and more contact, skin against skin.

In life, if you are present in your own body and conscious of your partner's, then you can relish each stage. I think one of the things I have learned about intimacy is to relish the moment, to resist end-gaming the encounter. It's wonderful just to enjoy a kiss for what it is, discovering the feeling of each other's lips, and then finally perhaps opening your mouth and including tongues in kissing. It is incredibly intimate to kiss with tongues; that might be the end of the encounter or the beginning of something more, but every moment of it is something to be appreciated and savored.

Yet it is only by learning to be grounded, by feeling ourselves rooted and present, and not distracted in any way, that this full sensual enjoyment can be unlocked.

THE EIGHT SILKEN MOVEMENTS

I was taught the Eight Silken Movements when I was training in On-Site Massage in the early 1990s and have incorporated them into my practice ever since. It is a simple and uplifting sequence of movements that helps you cultivate well-being in body, mind, and spirit.

The Eight Silken Movements have their roots in exercises first recorded 2,500 years ago and have been passed down through the centuries in China and beyond and have connections with traditional medicine. Like any physical sequence that has lasted so long, it has been developed as it has been passed down from practitioner to practitioner. What I'm sharing with you here is the sequence as I was taught it and also developed through my own practice.

There are many practitioners who can teach you their versions, either online or in person. There are also many beautiful videos of these practices available—please see the resources at the end of the book for one of my favorites. As you become familiar with these exercises, the intention is to perform them flowing from one to the next with a sense of silken ease.

The exercises are fundamentally standing exercises but can also be practiced sitting on a chair. They are also wonderful to practice outside in nature, allowing you to connect with the earth, the sky, and the beauty of nature

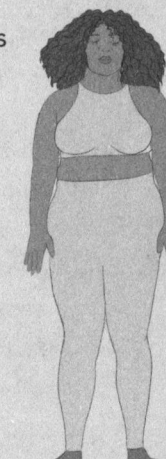

all around you, which will enhance your sense of calmness and connection.

I have suggested the flow of the inhale and the exhale for each exercise, but please explore for yourself the use of the breath with these silken movements.

1. Pressing up to the heavens with two hands

This exercise helps relieve tiredness and anxiety as well as insomnia.

- Start with your feet hip-width apart or sitting on a chair with your feet planted on the floor.

- Bring your hands in front of you and soften your elbows, fingertips toward each other, with your palms facing upward.

- Interlace your fingers together and on the in-breath draw up your hands until they reach your shoulder height, and then turn your palms upward and stretch your palms up toward the sky, keeping your fingers interlaced the whole time, holding up the sky with both hands.

- Exhale and release the fingers and extend the hands down to the sides as wide as possible and then let them come back down together with soft elbows, fingertips nearly touching and palms facing upward.

- Repeat this sequence three more times, connecting deeply with your breath each time.

2. Drawing the bow and letting the arrow fly

This exercise is excellent for opening the chest and increasing the lung capacity and also helping you to ground your lower body with a wide horse stance.

- Start by placing your feet in a wide stance as if you were riding a horse. Allow your knees to softly bend. If you are sitting on a chair, then you can open your legs out slightly beyond the width of the chair.

- Bringing the arms up in front of your chest with your left hand in front and your right hand behind, and then make your right hand into a fist as if holding a bowstring, and with your left hand hold your index finger pointing up toward the sky and curl your thumb and fingers in toward your palm.

- Inhale and extend your right hand and stretch out the right elbow as if pulling the bowstring while pushing the palm of the left hand out the side with the index finger pointing up toward the sky. Let your eyes follow the nail of your left index finger and enjoy the stretch right across the lungs as you complete the movement.

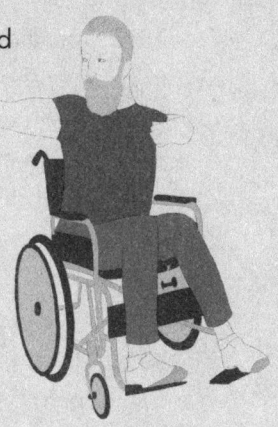

- As you exhale, let the left hand release so that both arms are extended outward at shoulder height, and let them fall back down before circling back up to the starting position, this time with your left hand behind and your right hand in front.

- Open the bow again, this time to the right side.

- Repeat this pair of movements two more times.

3. Separating heaven and earth

This exercise stretches the arms in opposite directions, pressing one palm up and one palm down. This exercise helps to support digestion.

- Stand with your feet shoulder-width apart and bring your arms in front of you, gathering your energy as you did with the first exercise.

- As you inhale, raise the left hand up the body and turn the palm upward above your head pressing the palm toward the sky. At the same time, take your right hand behind your back with your fingertips toward the center of the body and your palm

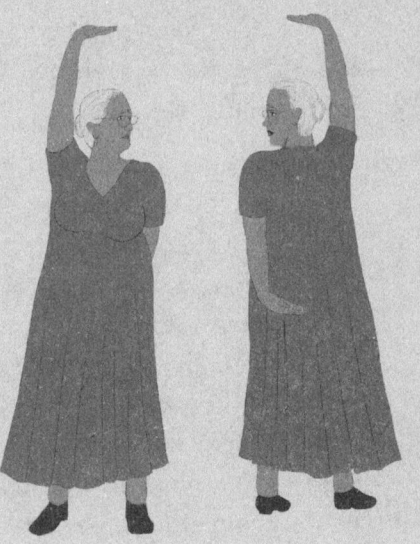

pressing down toward the ground, while looking over
your right shoulder.

- If you're sitting in a chair, you can just bring your right
hand to the side of you and press the arms in opposite
directions.

- As you exhale, circle your left hand back down toward
your starting position while releasing your right hand
and bringing it back in front of you.

- Repeat this sequence with your right hand reaching up
and your left hand pressing down with your gaze over
your left shoulder.

- Repeat this pair of movements two more times.

4. *Wise Owl gazes backward*

This is a wonderful exercise for opening the spine,
releasing stiff muscles, and improving your vitality, focus,
and energy levels.

- Stand with your feet shoulder-width apart, softening
your knees and bringing your hands up in front of your
chest with your right hand crossed behind your left
hand at the wrists.

- As you inhale, lower and pull open your arms down and
back on a diagonal line toward the ground, opening
your hands and stretching the fingers down toward the
earth while turning your chin over your left shoulder
and your gaze looking toward your left hand.

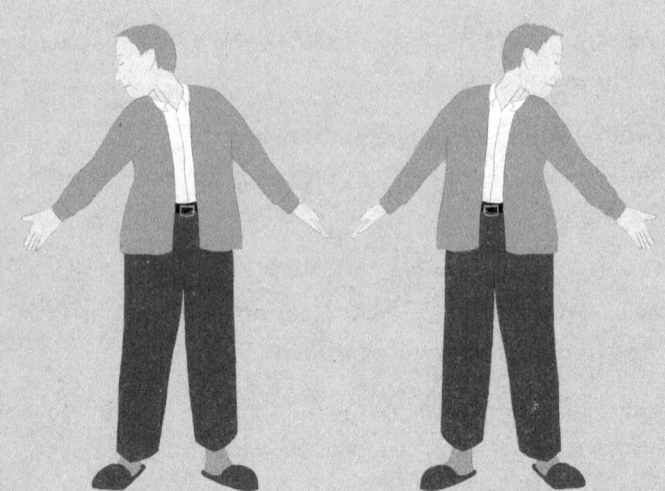

- As you exhale, soften your hands and knees, bringing your arms back in front of your chest, this time with your left hand behind and your right hand in front, ready to repeat the movement on the right side.

- Repeat both sides two more times.

5. Big Bear turns from side to side

This exercise is brilliant for releasing the lower back, and it helps support digestion and circulation.

- Stand with your legs in the horse-riding position, soften the knees and placing your hands on your hips or your waist, wherever it feels best for you.

- Breathe in to prepare and, as you exhale, bend your upper body from the waist over to the left.

- As you inhale, return to your upright starting position.

- As you exhale, bend your upper body from the waist over to the right.

- Inhale and return to your upright starting position.

- As you exhale, fold forward from the waist over the legs, going as far as is comfortable for you.

- Inhale and on the exhale roll yourself back up through the spine, stacking each and every vertebra until you are standing once more.

- Inhale and place your hands on your lower back or on your buttocks to support your spine, whatever is good for you, and then on the exhale gently stretch backward. If you have any back injuries, you may instead choose to adapt the move by simply lifting your gaze toward the sky or choose to leave this move out.

- Inhale and gently return to your upright starting position, ready to repeat, this time starting with the bend to the right side.

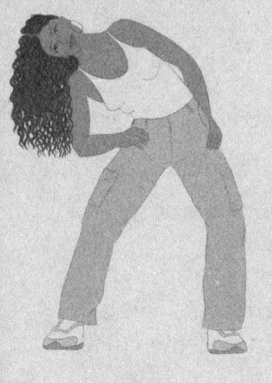
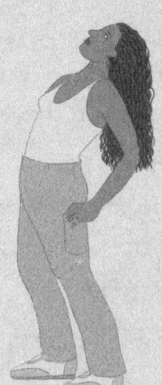
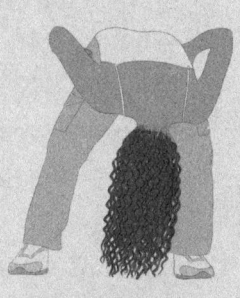

- Repeat this sequence two more times.
- Release the exercise by rolling your shoulders or moving your arms freely before moving on to the next silken movement.

6. Punching with an angry gaze

This exercise is wonderful for releasing pent-up energy, and it engenders courage and fortitude.

- Start by coming into the horse-riding stance with your legs wide and knees soft.
- Bring both your hands to your waist with curled fists and palms facing upward.
- Perform eight alternating punches facing forward, allowing yourself to flow from one movement to the next. Punch by extending your right hand forward, twisting your arm through the movement so that your palm is facing down at the end of the punch. Be mindful of gently squeezing the elbow as you extend the arm.
- You may wish to perform this movement vigorously, directing energy out of your "angry" eyes.
- If it is suitable, allow yourself to make whatever sound comes naturally with each punch, supporting the voice with a good belly breath.

- Once you have completed the eight punches forward, turn from your waist, keeping your feet anchored, face your left side and continue with eight more alternating punches.

- Then turn your torso from the waist to the right side and continue with eight more alternating punches.

- Inhale as you return to center and extend both hands out to the side, at shoulder height.

- On the exhale squeeze your arms down to your side while letting the air out of your body on a "shhh" sound.

- Take a moment of stillness to allow the energy to settle.

- Release the exercise by rolling your shoulders or moving your arms freely before moving on to the next silken movement.

7. Touching toes and bending backward

This exercise stretches the spine and increases the flexibility of the back, waist, and legs, helping give the body fresh energy.

- Start by standing in the horse-riding stance with your feet nice and wide and your knees gently softened.

- Breathe in to prepare, and exhale as you fold forward over the legs, bending as far as you can from the hips, reaching for the toes.

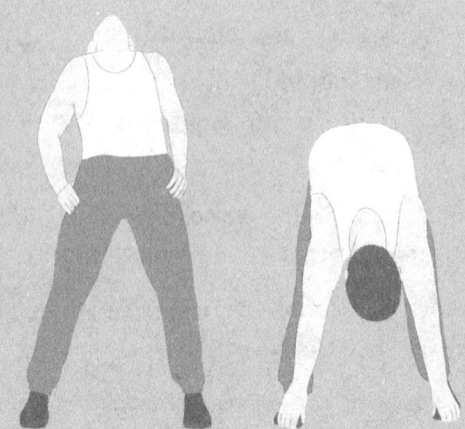

- If you can, place your hands underneath your toes or your feet, with the backs of your hands against the ground.

- Exhale and soften into the stretch, releasing and letting yourself hang over your legs stretching for three breaths. You may feel a stretch in your hamstrings.

- Then, on the next inhale, release the hands from the feet and as you exhale roll yourself back up through the spine, stacking each and every vertebra until you are standing once more.

- Inhale to prepare yourself, and on the exhale, gently continue into a backbend, placing your hands on your back to support your spine. If you have any back injuries, you may instead choose to adapt the move by simply lifting your gaze toward the sky or choose to leave this move out.

- Inhale, coming back to the center, and release your arms.

- Repeat this sequence two more times.

- Release the exercise by rolling your shoulders or moving your arms freely before moving on to the next silken movement.

8. Rising onto the toes

This is a great exercise that allows you to find your center and stillness. It enhances the body's balance and stability.

- Start by standing with your feet hip-width apart, with your hands down by your sides.

- Inhale to prepare and, as you exhale, rise up onto the balls of your feet, feeling as if there is a string at the top of your head pulling you up toward the sky.

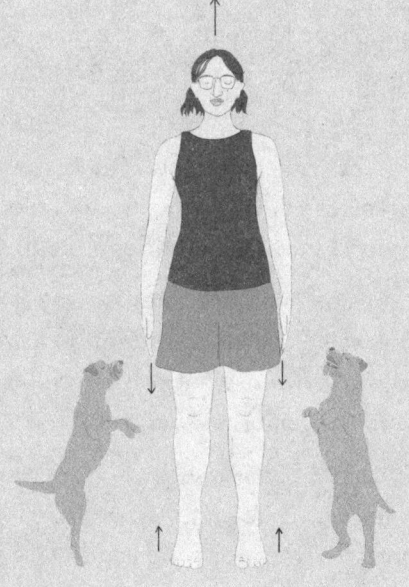

- At the same time, imagine there are strings pulling your hands down toward the earth through each and every finger.

- Inhale and allow your heels to come back down to the ground.

- On the exhale rise up again.

- Repeat this movement a third time; this time hold the balance, breathing as needed, and see if you can close your eyes and hold your balance.

- When you bring your heels down for the last time, release the movement by bending your knees and allowing a few gentle swings of your arms.

Relaxation to complete the Eight Silken Movements

After the Eight Silken Movements, it is good to complete your practice with a moment of stillness and calm, quiet relaxation.

- One way which you can do this is to lie down and allow yourself to release any energy you are holding down into the ground through eight deep breaths.

- If you are outside in nature, another way is to engage in a mindful walk, taking your attention to what you can hear, what you can see, what you can smell, what you can feel, and the textures around you.

- A third way is to hold a squatting position, feeling the release of the pelvis down to the earth, allowing your head to drop toward your hands and place the palms of your hands over your ears. Hold this position for eight breaths, enjoying the quiet and release.

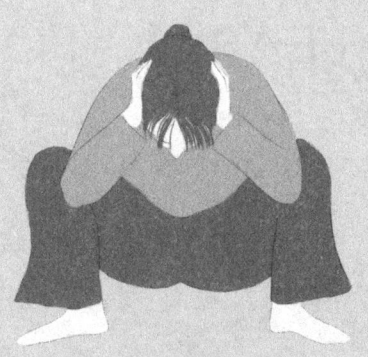

- When you have finished, come back to a standing position if that feels right for you, or come to lie on the floor for a few breaths.

- Whichever method you choose, take a moment to note how your body is feeling and reengage with whatever space you're in.

- Thank yourself for your practice and then set your intention for the next part of your day.

LEAPING FOOT

This is another exercise that focuses on the articulation of the feet, leading you through to a really joyous seated leap. Before you start, let's revisit the main points of weight in your feet, so you can understand how and what you're thinking of when you are anchoring your feet into the ground.

There are three main points of weight in your feet.

- Calcaneus: the center of your heel bone.

- Big toe joint: the head of metatarsal 1, where the big toe attaches to the foot.

- Little toe joint: the head of metatarsal 5, where the little toe attaches to the foot.

When standing or walking, the weight of the body is distributed across these three points. This tripod-like structure helps keep the foot stable and enables humans to stand, walk, and balance.

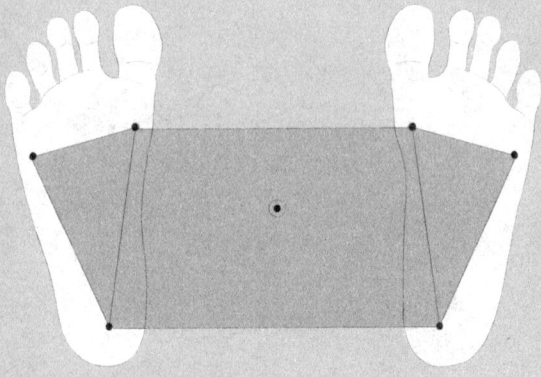

Now that you are visualizing these three points, you can begin the beautiful journey to a leap.

- For this exercise you will need a chair. Begin by sitting at the edge of the chair so that your feet can be flat on the ground, with your feet hip-width apart and your spine straight. Lightly hold on to the edge of the chair with your hands.

- Take a deep breath, and as you breathe out, imagine that you are sending roots down through the three points of connection: the center of the heel, the big toe joint, and the little toe joint. Imagining these roots can help you really feel that anchoring connection of the foot into the ground.

- You're just going to explore with the right foot first, so begin by anchoring your left foot into the ground.

- Lift the heel of the right foot. Come to the ball of the foot, pause for a moment, and then push up with the toes pointing, so it points to the ground while hovering just above it. Heel, ball, toe.

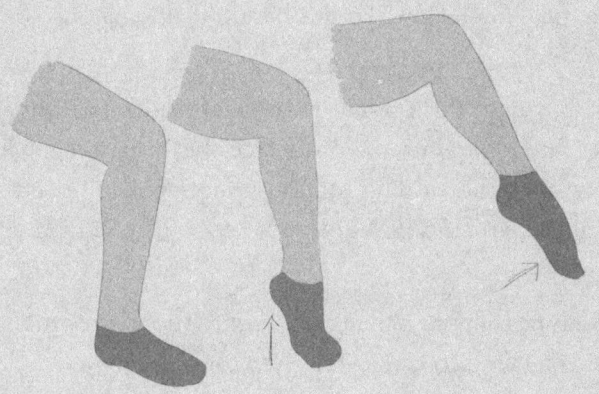

- Then reverse the movement, lowering your foot so the big toe connects with the earth, then rocking back to the ball of the foot and then lowering the heel. Landing toe, ball, heel. Feel your foot connected with the earth again.

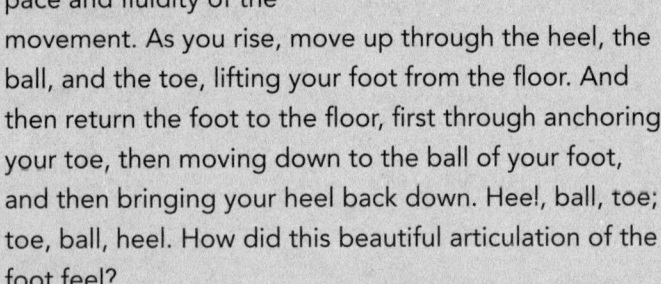

- You can now repeat this several times, experimenting with the pace and fluidity of the movement. As you rise, move up through the heel, the ball, and the toe, lifting your foot from the floor. And then return the foot to the floor, first through anchoring your toe, then moving down to the ball of your foot, and then bringing your heel back down. Heel, ball, toe; toe, ball, heel. How did this beautiful articulation of the foot feel?

- Next, repeat this on the other foot, with your right foot anchoring into the ground so that your left can lift. Heel, ball, toe landing toe, ball, heel. Notice how this might have felt different to the other foot: How did it feel?

- Come to stillness and allow the sensations to settle. You may wish to close your eyes for a moment.

- Now we've practiced with each individual foot, let's explore using both. How different might it feel to have both feet off the ground?

- You can hold on to the side of the chair for extra stability.

- It helps to stagger the feet so that one is slightly in front of the other.

- Starting with the left foot forward, right foot slightly pulled back, let's articulate both feet simultaneously: heel, ball, toe, and landing toe, ball, heel. Really enjoy that moment of suspension when both feet are in the air.

- Repeat this movement as many times as you like, exploring the pace and the fluidity of the movement. Notice how the movement feels through all the parts of your feet, parts you may not usually explore, and continue to breathe deeply as you move. Allow the inhale to find the moment of suspension before you come back to land again.

- Then swap to the right foot slightly forward, left foot pulled back, pushing off heel, ball, toe, and landing toe, ball, heel.

- Repeat this movement as many times as you like, exploring the pace and the fluidity of the movement. Notice how the movement feels through all the parts of your feet, parts you may not usually explore, and continue to breathe deeply as you move. How does it feel with the different foot leading? What is the same; what is different?

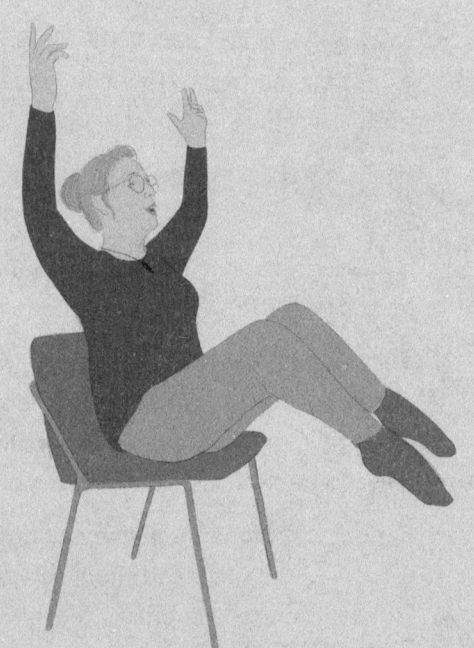

- As you progress, you may wish to take your hands off the chair: notice how different it might feel as you balance on your sit bones with both your feet in the air, enjoying that sensation of freedom.

- On your last articulation of the feet, pause at the 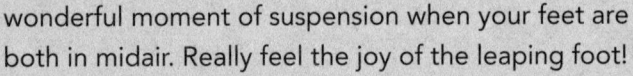 wonderful moment of suspension when your feet are both in midair. Really feel the joy of the leaping foot!

- As you lower your feet to the ground for the final time, take a moment to savor the energy through your body and feet.

- Now you have the option of coming to standing and exploring the sensation of the leap with three little jumps and a large final jump, going as high as you can, remembering to keep the articulation of the foot and enjoying the release and the excitement and elation that comes from the jump. Now you're ready to move on to the next part of your day.

CHAPTER SEVEN

CONNECTION AND COMMUNICATION

I think we all need to dance a bit more in life. When we first meet someone we like, we very often move with them, at a party or even just smooching on a balcony, in a garden, or on the street. Look at all the films where people fall in love as they fall into each other's arms or move in unison to the music. From Fred Astaire to *Lovers Rock* to the wonderful *We Live in Time*, where Florence Pugh's Almut and Andrew Garfield's Tobias fall off their feet in a romantic encounter, the image of someone being swept off their feet in movement is one of the great encouragements to intimacy onscreen.

It's no coincidence then that clubs are still places that people meet up. It's not just the atmosphere and the alcohol and the sense of fun, it's that these are spaces in which we can act out a ritual of engagement that goes beyond words. They are places where you can express your attraction to someone else in ways that don't involve sex; they are also environments where you can reveal something about yourself that isn't obvious in your everyday movements.

It's no coincidence either that *Strictly Come Dancing* in the UK and *Dancing with the Stars* in the US have become such popular shows. We love the voyeurism of seeing couples getting to know each other through dance; in part, we're admiring their artistry, but also there's a frisson of connection that goes beyond art. You watch the celebrities who are being taught to dance learn something new about themselves as they shed their inhibitions and begin to move.

Sometimes—in what's become known in Britain as the "curse of Strictly"—there is no distinction between the elation they feel with their partner at learning how to dance beautifully and the chemistry that lifts a dancing partnership into a sexual one. There have been affairs; there have been marriages. It's all down to the different sense of connection and communication you feel when you dance.

In my parents' time, this type of physical courtship was formalized. My parents met at the Irish Dances in Brixton; like other people of their generation, they still learned to ballroom dance and knew how to do a waltz or a foxtrot. Someone (usually a man) would ask someone else (usually a woman) to dance and would lead them by the hand to begin dancing with them. This was part of a historical pattern. Dancing with someone allowed you to gaze into their eyes, to touch each other, to play with each other within a formal frame.

If you are going to dance a waltz, you stand together and one partner puts their arm around a waist, the other puts their arm on a shoulder. The other hands are touching. The lead dancer's leg is between the other dancer's legs, and they pull their bodies together as they turn around. It is an intimate technique: you know the steps that you are going to dance, but there is a sense of exploration as well. Do I like having my body close to this person? Do they smell nice? How do they support me? Have they got spaghetti arms that are reaching places I would rather not be touched? Or have they got a strong frame? Do they move in time to the music in the same way that I do or are they dancing to a different rhythm? You discover so much about someone when you move with them—not least whether you wish to surrender to the dance with them.

This creation of intimacy through movement was part of a historical pattern. Villagers would leave the harvest and celebrate by flinging themselves in a roundel, a playful dance that enabled you to dance around someone, to bring your energy into contact with theirs. It was an official way to engage with someone else. In Elizabethan times, dancing was considered good exercise for the mind and body. Queen Elizabeth I practiced many styles of dance every day, and the upper classes would employ the most celebrated dancing masters to improve their standing at court. Being a good dancer boosted your status; you could show off your prowess and technique. By bowing in the prescribed way, the man put his leg forward, showing the shape of his calf. The better the dancer you were, the more shapely the calf, and therefore the more desirable you were as a catch for matrimony.

Look at the dancing scenes in *Shakespeare in Love*. Viola, the character Gwyneth Paltrow plays, uses formal dances to escape from her stuffy fiancé and build an intimacy with Shakespeare, in the shape of Joseph Fiennes. That film shows how the patterns and rhythms of dancing were the way that society created a formal journey for people to come to touch.

That journey continues down the centuries. In Jane Austen's *Pride and Prejudice*, filmed multiple times, Mr. Darcy meets his love Elizabeth Bennet at a ball. In the nineteenth century, codified dances such as the cotillion, waltz (daring!), polka, mazurka, and gallop added intricate embellishments and new improvisations to a system that allowed couples to meet and discover each other's bodies in a formal, regulated setting.

During the 1950s, rock 'n' roll maintained that structure, introducing a wilder way of moving, of lifts, flicks, and twists, alongside the hand-holding and intricate footwork. But by the sixties, a time of massive cultural shift, things began to change, as people danced opposite each other rather than with each other, doing their own thing to the music. The changing decades have brought different patterns: the rave culture of the 1990s triggered an upsurge in communal dancing, in search of a shared transcendence. However, by 2024, clubbing culture was on the decline, with more people dancing in front of a camera or watching other people dance on social media such as TikTok rather than going out to clubs and bars together.[1]

But in general, as dancing has become a form of self-expression and release rather than a partnership, we tend to underestimate dancing together as an intimate act.

Yet movement is a vital form of creating connection. To move and to dance is fundamental to who we are as humans. Through time, every Indigenous culture has danced. Every country expresses itself through its national dance. Dance fills the universe. Bees do a "waggle" dance to show the rest of the hive the site of the best flowers. Birds dance to attract a mate. Humans dance to worship their gods, to express their feelings—and to show off.

Everyone who has ever thrown some shapes on a dance floor knows that it's a way of meeting people and—just like the birds—making a move in the intricate process toward intimacy. It's a form of communication beyond words. In the late 1970s, the American dancer and musician Gabrielle Roth created an approach to movement known as the 5Rhythms, which remains hugely influential worldwide.[2] I was introduced to the thinking behind it by one of her pupils from her first ever training in 1982, Leo Rutherford, and I've found it very helpful in my life.[3] Broadly speaking, Roth focuses on five states of body movement, which are woven into a "wave." The first is flowing, which takes place on the in breath. It's here that the impulse and inspiration for movement is gathered.

Then there's staccato, which is an expulsion of power and energy out into the world. Flowing feels feminine, gentle, while staccato is all about the masculine; it's strong, intentional, and forceful. Staccato movement builds until it releases into chaos, the buffering of in and out breaths which clash and come together. It's like an orgasm, a culmination. As chaos falls away, you rediscover yourself in rhythm four, which is lyrical. This is the state where you dance your essence in that moment. Then that falls away to stillness, where everything ebbs away, and you feel yourself in the calm, and hear the silence, until a new inspiration takes hold, and the five rhythms of the wave begin again.

You have an idea, you think about it, you mull over it and make plans until you do something about it out in the world, which culminates in a crescendo of some sort: you either apply for a job and you've got it or ask someone out on a date and they say yes. There's the feeling that's left when that thing has been achieved, and then it falls away and you are ready for the next moment in your life or the next thing. The reason it's so brilliant is that you can apply the wave to anything. You can explore emotions through it—anger, jealousy, and love, for example. The very flow of a wave itself is like an act of intimacy, of coming together, rising in passion, through to orgasm, the postcoital glow, and the stillness and peace in the aftermath of that orgasm.

I really suggest you try to dance in this way. There are 5Rhythms sessions held across the globe, so you can join a class and learn the technique to use alone, with a partner, with a friend, with a community. But in general, as you journey through the wave, you eventually fall into stillness before the rhythm starts again. And if you repeat the motion, over three waves, for example, you suddenly drop into the body, into that place of otherness beyond your head. There is something in the body's wisdom that is beyond the hold of the mind that gives freedom to explore exciting possibilities. The movement actually takes you somewhere else. Roth expanded this into the idea of a moving meditation, where you set an intention and then just dance your way through it. You are moving things through the body and allowing thoughts to be freed. Just as you might go for a massage to soothe a sore muscle when there is some kind of physical trauma trapped in your body, so dancing thoughtfully in this way allows you to release a memory or a thought or an emotion that is locked inside you. Roth devised this dynamic movement practice to take people beyond their limitations, "to ignite creativity, connection and community."[4]

The way you express yourself in this dance is entirely open; each individual finds their own means of expression, whether it is a young person who can move with ease or a person who uses a wheelchair who might just move their head and their little finger. The structure gives focus and shape, but there is complete freedom within it. You let the music play, and you let your body respond. One day you might have huge amounts of energy and fling yourself around the room; on another day, you might just lie on the floor and feel yourself through the rhythm. In this place, you often discover something exciting and beyond what you have thought of before.

I have always been struck by the revelatory qualities of movement. When actors choose something with their mind, it can be quite conventional, but discovering something that they feel with their bodies can take them on more exciting paths. It's remarkably similar in intimate relationships. You can understand a lot about how someone feels about you from how they hold themselves in relation to you. Instinctively you tend to explore this physically; you get out of your own way and let the body do the talking! This is why when people first meet, on a dance floor or elsewhere, they often unconsciously mirror each other's movements. We want to show we are one with the other person, that our bodies and our minds are in unison. We'll sit like them, move like them. Verbally we will say we are interested in the same things as them (even if it isn't entirely true). We establish images and feelings of harmony. Interestingly, understanding mirroring can be used consciously to alter the mood of a situation. If you want to encourage someone to engage more honestly with you, then you might think about actively opening up your body to them, breathing slowly, inviting a conversation.

If you sit as if you are wound up, and all your muscles are tight, then the person you are meeting with might read your pose as showing you are upset and closed off. In conflict resolution, body language is part of the training. If someone is upset, the training advises that you don't try to match them—but try to act expansively, taking full breaths, lowering your voice, so that you are not meeting but dissipating their emotion. You invite them back into their breath. It shows you've seen the dynamic, that you understand their agitation. It enables them to feel seen and understood.

This is what we want in our intimate relationships too. Communicating properly springs from getting on to the other person's wavelength. There is no point in you deciding that you are going to have a lovely romantic evening, dimming the lights, lighting the candles, cooking dinner, and then, when your partner walks in, not noticing that they are exhausted because they have had a terrible day at work. You can't just offer and then expect someone to be present as soon as they walk in the door. It's a question not just of offering but of leaving a space for the other person to respond.

In films, people are very often walking into rooms, pulling a loved one into a clinch, and immediately the embraced person will be ready and responsive for intimacy. In life, if your partner puts their arms around you in the kitchen at the end of a long day and starts thrusting against you on the tabletop, you might enjoy it and agree to their initiation of sex, but you're just as likely to feel it's entirely the wrong moment and push them away instead of succumbing to passion.

One of the keys to a successful relationship is under-standing the other person's perspective and working together to create something you both value. When we are in the first throes of passion—the sort that is so well represented in terms of what we see on TV and film—then lust takes over. There's a sexual drive where you just can't wait to be together. It's as much about your own lust and your own sexual drive as about being turned on by the other person.

It's when this kind of passion is spent that relationships begin to develop and require some tending. That is the moment when you truly look at each other and start to explore deeper ways of communicating. Sitting side by side next to each other on the sofa watching TV may become the principal activity that you share with your partner—but if you reach out your hand and hold theirs, it can still be a form of intimacy. It is doing something together in order to spend time with each other.

Creating these spaces for communication and connection become more important. Intimacy is not—whatever we might like to think—always spontaneous. In fact, it very rarely is.

That is why sex and relationship counselors such as Linsey Blair, often advocate scheduling a time for intimacy, making a space where you can be together and explore your relationship. I first met Blair in 2020 and have worked with her ever since. She teaches the anatomy of sexual arousal and dysfunction to the practitioners I have trained and, as a fully accredited sex and relationship therapist, offers valuable advice on improving and deepening the depiction of intimacy onscreen. I have come very much to trust her advice and guidance. Blair is very clear that regularly agreeing to a date on your calendar where you can be together with your partner or prospective partner to give time and space to explore your relationship is a vital part of intimacy. The period you set aside for this may or may not lead to sex. But it is precious whatever the outcome.

Couples are very often reluctant to do this, thinking that it will take the spontaneity out of their relationship, and that there is something clinical and forced about making time for one another in this way. Blair has a ready answer for that. "Couples come to me because they are not having sex, so this idea of spontaneity clearly isn't working. You schedule watching a film on Netflix. You say, let's make time on Wednesday to see this thing that we both want to see. Most tasks and activities require some conversation and planning. Yet people expect sex to happen in the moment. That just doesn't make sense, especially when couples are going to bed at different times and getting up at different times. Especially when they have got kids. There's not much couple time left in the world when you've got children and you're working full-time jobs. You have to make time to be together, and make it special, inviting, and intimate. Not boring or routine."

Carving out time to spend with someone is inherently caring; it shows that you've invested in your relationship, and you are putting the other person first. You might want to try to create a more intimate space than is usual in your day-to-day living, perhaps changing the lighting or having music playing to make it more special. You might want to go out together. You might decide to have a regular date night, for example. Or a conversation before bed every night. The important thing is that this creation of a place where you can be intimate works for you and nurtures your intimacy.

It is another myth that simple proximity will bring

people together. When Covid swept the world and people were trapped in their houses during lockdown, there was a lot of speculation in newspapers that it would lead to a baby boom. In fact, the opposite proved true. Analysis of live birth rates in 24 European countries showed that birth rates declined by an average of 14.1 percent during the nine months after the first wave of Covid-19 lockdowns. Only after that did birth rates begin slowly to recover. The findings, compiled by the Human Fertility Database, were fairly consistent in most of the countries studied: down by 12.2 percent in Belgium, 14.4 percent in France, 17.2 percent in Italy, 23.5 percent in Spain, and 13 percent in the UK. In Sweden, which did not introduce a lockdown, there was no decline in live birth rates.[5]

The researchers argue that there is no single reason for the decline. Factors may include people deciding to postpone conception because of worry about the state of the world, or an overwhelmed health service. But it is also possible that the actual fact of being locked down together meant some couples were less likely to procreate. "I remember thinking how little people understood about sexuality if they thought that birth rates would rise because everyone was together in the same house," Blair says. "Couples tend to stop having sex when their partner becomes part of the routine."

In thinking about nurturing intimacy, it's important to recognize that male and female attitudes are very different. In *Gentleman Jack,* which is about love and sex between women, the intimate scenes were written to reflect women's experience, which is much more focused on the emotional connection, being seen and loved by their partner, inviting a more inward, slower build to intimacy. It told the story of the life of Anne Lister, the English diarist who lived in the late eighteenth and early nineteenth centuries and is often referred to as "the first modern lesbian." As intimacy coordinator, I worked closely with the expert historian Anne Choma, reading Lister's words and honoring the quality of her love with different partners and her explorations of self-pleasure.

I also consulted people from the queer community and researched books, particularly *The Whole Lesbian Sex Book*, which was first published in 1999 with the aim of offering "information and encouragement for all women who desire women," covering topics such as exploring personal desires and fantasies, how masturbation improves sex, and how to achieve the preferred orgasm.[6]

When I was researching the creation of intimate encounters for *It's a Sin*, on the other hand, a series by Russell T Davies about the lives and sexual encounters of a group of friends during the HIV/AIDS crisis of the 1980s, my focus was on providing authenticity in the portrayal of queer male sexuality. I've also worked on similar scenes in *Sex Education* and *I May Destroy You*.

In each case, I've realized that men tend to be more visually and physically driven when it comes to who they find attractive, and so have found ways of showing this in the approach to sexual encounters. As for the choreography, it's important that the physicality of the positions are accurate, so I researched body shapes and possible positions in Axel Neustädter's *Gayma Sutra* and talked to people from the gay community to make sure we got it right.[7] On *It's a Sin*, it was particularly joyous to work on a set where the director and most of the cast were from the queer community so they could help bring detail to the choreography.

Authentic representation is important particularly for marginalized communities. A blog by Tessa Kaur makes the point that it helps to "combat stereotypes and ignorance." She quotes a 2015 study, which found that "when straight people are more exposed to gay characters on TV they become more accepting of gay equality." On top of that, a 2020 survey by GLADD, the world's largest LGBTQ+ media advocacy organization, and Procter & Gamble found that queer representation increased queer acceptance by up to 45 percent.[8]

I'd like to begin to have more conversations with filmmakers, writers, directors, and performers to invite consideration of how intimate scenes are written in order to show the importance of different kinds of intimacy. One of the reasons that *Normal People* made such an impact was its reality in depicting the narrative of the sexual encounters. The postcoital scenes were touching and truthful; they showed something that people could relate to and understand. They also underlined the fact that it is the entire encounter that is important in intimate relationships. They made postcoital tenderness and relaxation sexy. They were important to making sex onscreen more relevant to our intimate lives.

Nurturing these feelings in our lives and with our lovers is a way of deepening and preserving intimacy. Connection is incredibly important. The influential movement director Trish Arnold devised a movement exercise, which I often use, called the Swing (see the box on page 213). Arnold was a pioneer of movement training for actors and worked with the British theatrical innovator Joan Littlewood among others. Her system of pure movement work enabled actors to develop a sense of impulse and connection to breath by devising—and I am quoting the *Guardian* obituary here—"a methodology and approach that worked from impulse (initial mental, emotional and physical responses) and release (letting go of habits of movement), so that actors could adopt the physical signals that help an audience recognize a character on stage or screen."[9]

With the Swing, Arnold encouraged actors to swing their arms forward on the out breath, experiencing the hiatus, the charged moment of suspension, before gravity took the swing back on the in breath, allowing momentum to take them on a sweep of the arm that slows as it reaches the top of the gravitational pull behind the body. At that second, there's this amazing pause, before the swing releases back down and begins its arc again.

When I was learning to act, because of my dyslexia, I always found that learning the text was hard, and so I would tend to hold on to the words in the script and the thought, gathering my intention to myself, making sure I did not forget them, or trying to show that I knew the lines, rather than really being in relationship with the words. There was no relation between language and the breath. I didn't trust my connection to remembering the words, so I didn't communicate. Arnold's techniques helped me to overcome that. If you want to communicate properly, there has to be a call and then a response, an in breath and an out breath. You send your words into a place of not knowing and pause to allow the words to land.

In the pause, you don't know how your words will be accepted by someone else, or what they are going to say next. On the in breath, you are allowing time and space for the other person's words to affect you; on the out breath, you are sending words back to them so that they can react to what you have said. Onstage, this makes communication more naturalistic. It develops the energy and action of the actor being in their body, trusting inspiration, and letting character emerge. Like Gabrielle Roth's 5Rhythms, it is a technique that lets you get out of your own way.

In life, this is just as true: you can't be in a relationship, intimate or otherwise, if you're held in and not letting your breath move freely. It means you are not being present; you are not really listening. The dynamic of the Swing is about what you are sending out into the world—that woosh of breath and your body moving forward—and after a moment of leaving yourself undone in the hiatus, then really receiving something from someone on the in breath.

If you felt like doing it with a partner, it would have positive benefits. It fills your lungs with breath, it wakes up the body and allows it to fill the space. It is also essentially freeing. As children, most of us love going up on a swing. There's something in our psyche that responds to the excitement of the movement, of the air rushing past as we go up and down. As we let our arms swing forward and backward, the mental image of a swinging body helps us to imagine the to and fro that is required in proper communication and connection. Nowhere is this more important than in the space where we cultivate our intimate relationships.

If we go back to that scene in the kitchen where one partner grabs the other, expecting intercourse, and the other isn't ready, the exercise of the Swing explains why. There's no offer, no chance for pause and return. One person is in the mood but hasn't checked that the other feels the same—and hasn't given a space, a breath, for them to return the offer or make a different one that preserves the mood but takes it in a different direction. This failure to read a partner's needs is an inhibitor in developing intimacy. It might be the case that instead of kissing and cuddling, what you really need to do is dance together to the music that is playing while you cook— leaving space and time for a reaction. Or perhaps on this occasion a bit of a dance might be enough. A little dance where you kiss and cuddle in time to the music is a fantastic thing to do. In fact, the kitchen is the place where my partner and I dance the most!

Yet the other thing I have learned from life, as much as movement practice, is that intimacy thrives in space as well as in proximity. I am always a bit anxious when couples tell me that they have never spent a night apart since they met. It seems to me that part of a healthy relationship is giving people room to be themselves apart from you, as well as with you. Linsey Blair reports that it is often the moment when a woman sees her husband carrying their child upstairs or glimpses him across a crowded room that triggers interest. Seen up close, the picture is routine. From afar, sparks begin to fly.

This again is the pattern of the Swing. Connection and communication are often about movement—toward someone, or away from something. This is not a static thing. Part of foreplay is literally getting into sync with someone else's energy. Once you wake up the space between each other and that intimate dance with a partner, then you can take a relationship into a sensuous encounter. That's the subject of the next chapter.

SWING

This exercise has two sequences. The first is forward-facing, in which your arms will draw the shape of a wheel. This allows you to experience momentum and a sense of weight and suspension. The second is a horizontal swing that allows you to feel your body expand from fingertip to fingertip and inhabit your space across your chest.

Arm swings loosen and stretch the muscles and joints in your shoulders, back, and neck, help to improve circulation, and are a great way to enhance shoulder mobility, range of motion and stability. Enjoy the momentum and exhilaration of the freedom of the swing.

Wheel Swing

- Start by standing straight in a neutral stance, with your feet hip-width apart, and then raise both arms above your head in a fluid motion with your palms facing toward you, pulling your elbows in toward each other, with your gaze following your hands.

- To begin the Swing, softly bend your knees, allowing your arms to sweep down to your sides.

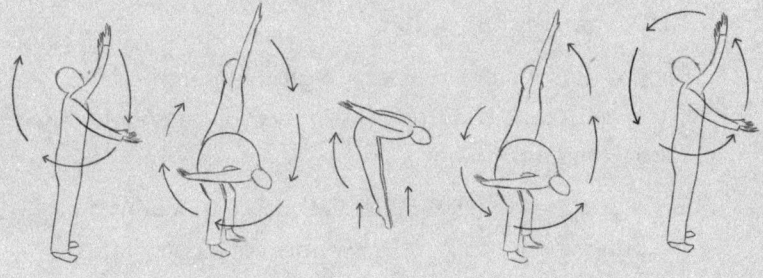

- Keeping your core engaged for stability, continue the movement of your arms flowing behind you, lifting them up above your head as if you were preparing to dive into a swimming pool.

- Continuing the fluid movement in a great circle, bending at the waist and stretching your fingertips forward, folding your body down and bringing your stomach onto your thighs (or as far as is comfortable for you to bend forward), so that your fingertips brush the floor, continuing their circle up behind you, holding in a moment of suspension, head toward the floor.

- This completes the first half of the Swing.

- In a fluid movement, release your arms back down to the floor, soften your knees, stretch the arms forward as they rise up above your head, straighten your knees, and come back up.

- Engaging your core for stability as your arms circle behind you, soften the knees and allow the arms to swing forward, bringing the elbows in toward each other, palms facing toward you as you complete the Swing with your hands above your head and your gaze following your hands.

- This completes one Swing.

- Repeat the whole movement, eight times, at first slowly but then gradually getting faster as your body gets used to the movement.

- Once you are comfortable with the Swing, an option is to continue onto four more swings that incorporate a jump as the arms sweep behind you with your body folded over your legs.

- On either the eighth or the twelfth Swing (depending on whether or not you feel like jumping today), catch your arms above your head and stop, looking up at your palms for a moment.

- To complete the exercise, lift the arms above the head and open them to the sides, releasing the arms back to a neutral standing position.

- Take a breath to recenter yourself before starting the next Swing sequence.

Horizontal Swing

- Start by widening your stance to shoulder-width and slowly open your arms out to the side, bringing them to shoulder height, palms facing down. Keep your core engaged and maintain an upright posture.

- Prepare on an inhale and on the exhale, soften your knees, and allow the arms to drop back in toward your body, bringing your arms to cross in front of you.

- As you inhale, release the arms back out to shoulder height, stretching the fingers away in opposite directions, enjoying the feeling of width and expansion across the chest into space.

- On the exhale, bring your arms back in again to cross in front of you and on the inhale release them back out to the side.

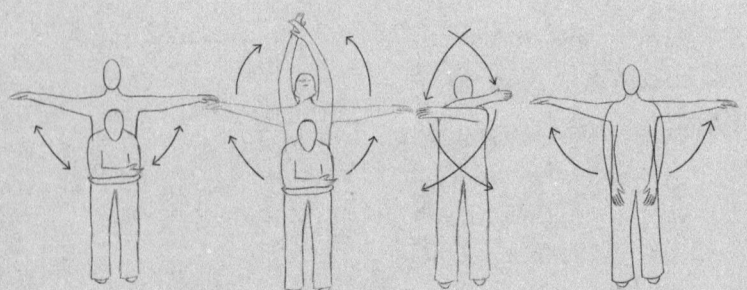

- Repeat this movement three times.
- On the fourth Swing, releasing the arms across the body, allow the momentum to lift your arms all the way up over your head, opening out to the side and continuing in a full circle until they cross in front of your body again.
- This completes the first half of the Swing.
- For the second half, inhale and release the arms out to shoulder height as before, exhaling to bring them in again across the body.
- Repeat this three times.
- On the fourth Swing, allow the momentum to carry your arms out and up above your head in a great circle and continue down in front of your body and lifting out to the side at shoulder height once more.
- This completes the full horizontal Swing sequence, ready to repeat once more.
- When you have completed the whole horizontal Swing sequence twice, soften your arms and come back to a neutral stance.

- Come back to standing hip-width apart, and to stillness.

- Close your eyes and take a moment to connect with how you feel.

- When you have given yourself enough time to reflect on the exercise, open your eyes if they are not already open, and bring yourself back into the space.

- If it works for you, a good way to anchor your experience is to write any thoughts or reflections in a notebook or to draw any images, shapes, and colors that came to you.

CHAPTER EIGHT

THE MYTH AND REALITY OF SEXUAL AROUSAL

When intimacy is portrayed authentically onscreen, it isn't just women who benefit. It can be a revelation for male partners, the starting point for powerful conversations about having better, more connected sex. Emma Thompson noticed something similar after her groundbreaking mirror scene in *Leo Grande*. It started conversations on difficult topics. She told Caitlin Moran in *The Times* that some of the most interesting reactions had been from male viewers "young and old, having, maybe for the first time, conversations about female sexual pleasure. One older man said he saw the film and immediately went home and started to talk to his wife about what might give her pleasure. For the first time."[1]

I know I talk a lot about what we see onscreen. That's partly because it is my profession. But it is also because what we see is closely connected to how we feel and unless we start to change the conversation and alter the view, then our own intimate lives will suffer. After we met at the

Sundance Film Festival, the psychoanalyst Dr. Orna Guralnik told me: "What's portrayed onscreen is often the benchmark for how things are supposed to be. When they're talking about intimate relations, [people] don't turn to the Bible. They turn to Hollywood."

As I've said over and over again, what we see onscreen is based on a myth rather than reality. The myth, or fantasy if you like, can make people feel good or bad about themselves. But it will very often distance them from their authentic experience. Dr. Orna pointed to one couple who appeared on her hugely popular TV show *Couples Therapy* in which the woman confessed that she had real difficulties with the idea of what she called "Tuesday sex."

Tuesday sex is the kind of weekday sex that establishes a connection with a partner, an intimacy that preserves your relationship and feels part of your routine rather than something mind-blowing and special. Tuesday sex is incredibly valuable and important in a committed relationship in cementing a regular connection and strengthening emotional ties. Yet Tuesday sex is rarely depicted in mainstream Hollywood, which opts very often for erotic intimacy, such as the scenes depicted in *9½ Weeks* or *Magic Mike's Last Dance.* "That's the kind of fantasy Hollywood has produced forever, and yet it would be great if Hollywood could get interested in that kind of sex [i.e., Tuesday Sex]," Dr. Orna told me. "As opposed to Disney World sex, for example. It could be tremendously good for people to be located in the reality of their own body, and their partner's body, not mediated through all of these super fantasies about what is supposed to happen. They are actually distancing."

This is precisely what worries me. In the real world, in real relationships, people's lives are fundamentally filled with Tuesday sex. It's the same when you go to see a play. Nine times out of ten, you might just vaguely enjoy it—and then once in a while, it will absolutely hit the spot. You experience something sensational. We need to acknowledge that that is the case. I would say that, particularly in long-term relationships, if you're lucky enough to be with someone who wants Tuesday sex, and you continue to have it, then you should be celebrating. If you are carrying on a relationship with a long-term partner, then the fact that either of you wants to be intimate on a regular basis should be a cause for joy. You don't need bells and whistles to make it special. If couples of all genders embrace Tuesday sex, we're on our way to a better understanding of intimacy.

I had a friend who made it a policy always to have sex when their partner offered because—she reasoned—her lover might not be asking in another 10 years' time, and she didn't want to miss a single opportunity. She stood by this plan even when she wasn't in the mood for intimacy at first, because she felt it was important to maintain an active intimate life. The result was one of the happiest relationships I have ever seen.

Yet we simply don't see enough Tuesday sex onscreen— those moments when a loving couple come together in a way that isn't earth-shattering or fantastic, or marked with swelling music and soft lighting, but instead actually suggests that two people who love each other might want to be intimate together in an everyday setting. It's rare to see those moments, though shows such as Sharon Horgan's *Catastrophe*, where the comedy was built around a married couple coping with the arrival of young children in their lives, had a truthfulness that felt special.

It's clear to me that men, just as much as women, need a change in the stories that we are telling ourselves. The crisis in masculinity, which is an accepted part of early-twenty-first-century life, means that our boys and men are desperate for role models they can aspire to. With the amount of fighting and aggression we see onscreen, you really feel for men who want to be gentle and kind, or those who are perhaps struggling with their mental health or striving to find their place in the world.

Yet so much of modern cinema offers unhelpful templates of being. If women are too often shown as victims, men are regularly depicted as predators and murderers, sociopaths on the prowl to destroy. At the other extreme, they are Marvel-style heroes, invincible and untouched by feelings. Marvel supermen are so busy saving the world that they don't have time to engage in love and relationships.

Nick Schager in an article in *Esquire* in 2021 is one of those commentators to note that "the Marvel Cinematic Universe is sexually dysfunctional." He goes on to argue: "The studio's cultural hegemony has given birth to a contemporary cinematic landscape of distinctly un-erotic blockbusters, that largely eschew sex altogether, the better to appeal to their teen target audiences. That those kids might want to see incredibly good-looking movie stars having adult relations seems to be beside the point; innocent virtue allows the studio to peddle its product to the largest number of domestic and international consumer markets possible, not only in movie theaters but on toy shelves and clothing racks. Such business objectives trump everything else."[2]

In a sharply written piece in the digital magazine *Blood Knife*, R S Benedict went further. "Actors are more physically perfect than ever: impossibly lean, shockingly muscular with magnificently coiffed hair, high cheekbones, impeccable surgical enhancements and flawless skin, all displayed in form-fitting superhero costumes with the obligatory shirtless scene thrown in to show off shredded abs and rippling pecs . . . Even background extras are good-looking, or at least inoffensively bland. No one is ugly. No one is really fat. Everyone is beautiful. And yet, no one is horny. Even when they have sex, no one is horny. No one is attracted to anyone else. No one is hungry for anyone else."[3]

This is a relatively recent development. Christopher Reeve's Superman had plenty of time to fly through the air holding hands with his love Lois Lane while still saving the planet from extinction. It was only in 2002 that Kirsten Dunst's Mary Jane gently kissed Tobey Maguire's Spiderman while he was hanging upside down on a building. But though, in the hands of Tom Holland 's Peter Parker and Zendaya's MJ, Spiderman is still the tenderest of the Marvel genre, as the twenty-first century has progressed, the hard-plated armor superheroes wear seems to extend to their bodies and their hearts as well. The focus is on how they can fight and how they can defend themselves, and their sense of vulnerability and intimacy has vanished.

When it comes to their intimate lives, men are just as much a victim of cinematic myths as women. On the one hand, they have action figures, honed and invulnerable. On the other, as I've said before, it is clear that the easy availability of online pornography has become a major issue. Even in mainstream imagery, the vocabulary of filmmaking causes confusion. It's worth bearing in mind here just how close some of the assumptions of pornography and mainstream depictions of sex have become. Pornography is explicit, yet the images of intimacy we often see on TV and in the films do nothing to challenge its narrative.

Hollywood might not screen sex scenes that last 20 minutes, but it does assert that from desire to penetration, sex is extremely fast, an erection is instant and lasts, a woman enjoys that kind of intimacy and will come to orgasm. Too many sex scenes subtly confirm pornography's patterns, creating the misleading impression that spontaneous and instant penetration is possible for men—and pleasing for most women. This is simply not true. The erotic life of women tends to be tied to their emotional life. Intimacy arises from an emotional and psychological connection. The anatomy of arousal for men and for women is also utterly different.

In this respect, my work with Linsey Blair has been eye-opening. The first time I met Blair, I was already working as an intimacy coordinator. I was in my mid-50s. Yet her detailed descriptions of the cycles of male and female anatomy, shown in a presentation given by her, and presented on the pages that follow, were a revelation to me and gave me a completely different understanding of male and female sexual anatomy. This understanding of the anatomy and cycle of men and women's arousal deepened my understanding of what I could present onscreen, and what people experience offscreen. This information is something that ideally everyone (not just intimacy coordinators) would benefit from being taught, so that it can be incorporated in our relationships with our bodies, our sexual lives, and our sexual partners.

As the drawings accompanying this chapter show, arousal for men and women follows different patterns. The male response cycle is a linear journey of desire, excitement, plateau, orgasm, and resolution. You can think of this akin to a journey up a mountain and back again.

1. Excitement   2. Plateau

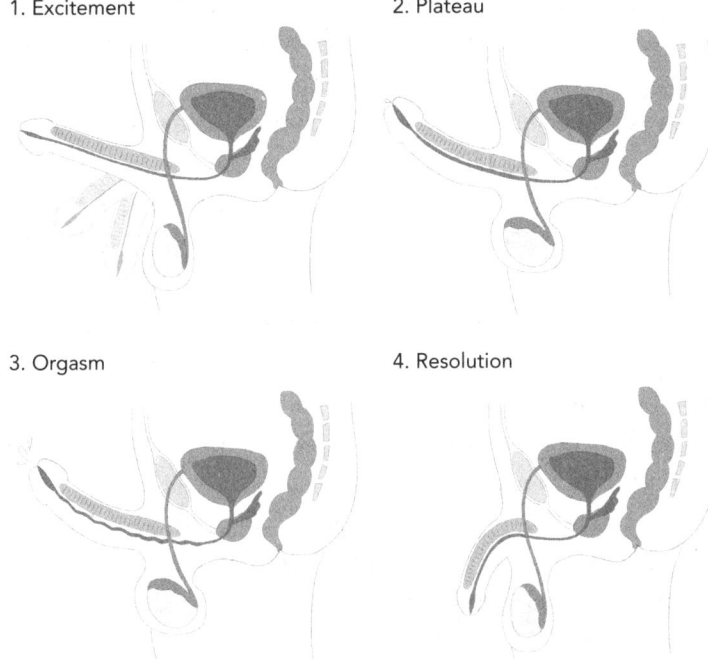

3. Orgasm   4. Resolution

The female response cycle is circular, starting with a willingness to be receptive, initiation of desire through appropriate sexual stimuli, arousability that leads to high arousal and responsive desire, through to orgasm and resolution. Desire in women is not linear and is likely to be spontaneous only when they are fertile. Often it arrives quite late in the buildup to orgasm.

Knowing that the cycles of arousal for men and women

have such different shapes is vital in giving us a key to the fundamental experience of male and female sexual encounters. Knowing the detail of the difference in libidos helps to understand what is happening and explains a physicality that has nothing to do with whether and how you love somebody, but rather to understand that, as Blair said in our interview for this book, "it takes longer for women to 'get into' sex than men; this is not low libido, it is different libido" and "because of the difference in libidos, 'good sex,' i.e., sex that is mutually enjoyable, needs to have a lot more female foreplay so that she can 'get in.'"

It's no wonder that when I asked Blair what was the most misleading intimate myth that she sees onscreen, she laughed and said she didn't really know where to start. "But I guess speed. Which is complicated because that's so difficult to show onscreen. The majority of sexual pain in women comes from the fact that they are penetrated too early. They don't have enough foreplay. They are not using lubricant. It is a massive point of sexual education for everyone to understand that it generally takes women about 20 minutes to be ready for penetration, yet what tends to be depicted is a couple kissing and then penetrating within less than five minutes."[4]

I realize that no one wants to watch a sex scene that lasts half an hour and consists mainly of foreplay. But there are ways to suggest the engagement in foreplay and the need for lubrication: I can choreograph a scene that shows the use of lubricant or indicates a little extra foreplay. One reason people relate to that first intimate encounter between Connell and Marianne in *Normal People* is that it does actually suggest that penetration only happens when she is aroused and ready.

The speed of the female orgasm that is often depicted—within five minutes of penetration—is another damaging myth. A lot of women don't have an orgasm via penetration, relying on clitoral stimulation to bring them to climax. We do sometimes see this on film. But more often than not, a woman is shown reaching orgasm very quickly and in positions that are likely to be uncomfortable, even painful and unsatisfying. Mutual, spontaneous orgasm, which is another film trope, is a rare phenomenon because male and female cycles of desire are so different.

In order to achieve vaginal orgasm, a woman's internal clitoris needs to be activated. The clitoris is a little-understood Y-shaped organ that has as much arousal tissue as the penis and can get as engorged as a penis. The difference is that the majority of the organ is internal.

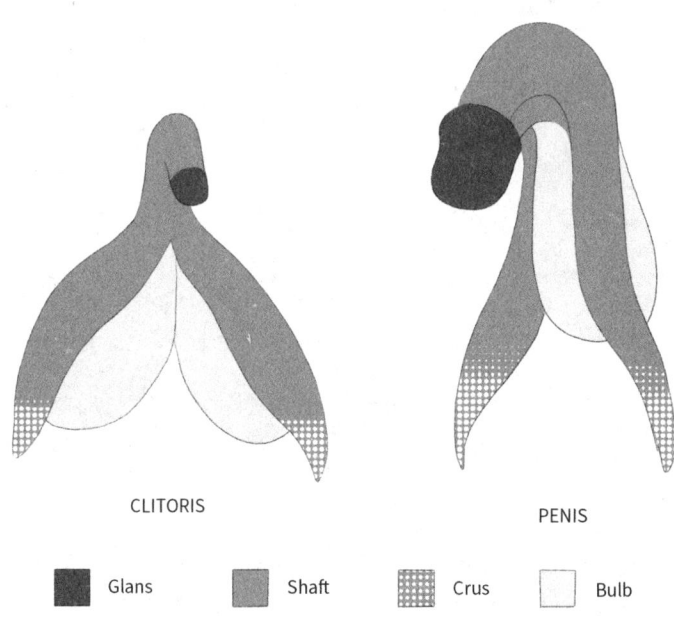

CLITORIS

PENIS

Glans   Shaft   Crus   Bulb

In an unaroused state, the uterus is relaxed and low, leans over the bladder, and is eggplant-shaped, with the vaginal walls lying close together.

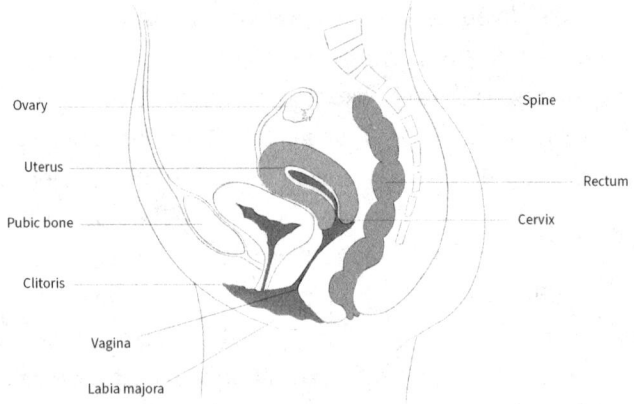

Here are illustrations of all of the following stages, based on a presentation given to me by Linsey.

In the excitement phase:

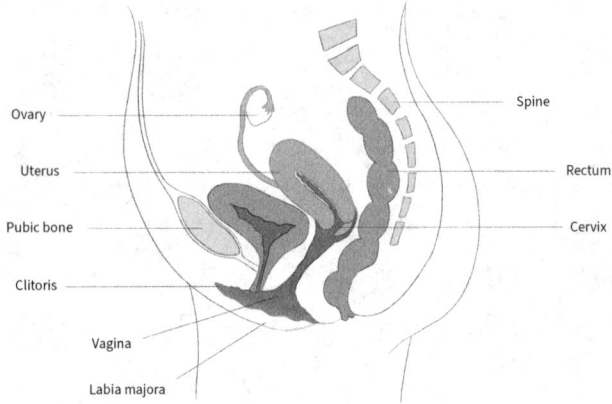

- *Vaginal lubrication is produced within 10–20 seconds of sexual stimulation.*

- *The vagina lengthens and distends, and the uterus begins to elevate.*

- *The inner and outer vaginal lips become engorged with blood and increase in size.*

- *The clitoris may become erect and is extremely sensitive to touch.*

- *The vagina is insensitive to touch.*

- *A "sex flush" appears over the breasts and chest; the breasts swell, and the nipples become erect.*

- *Breathing becomes heavier; the heart rate and blood pressure increase.*

As a woman, you don't have to be fully aroused to be lubricated enough to enjoy penetrative sex, but it will be more pleasurable as the body moves into the plateau phase when the vagina is opening up and the uterus is ascending in preparation for potential orgasm.

In the plateau phase:

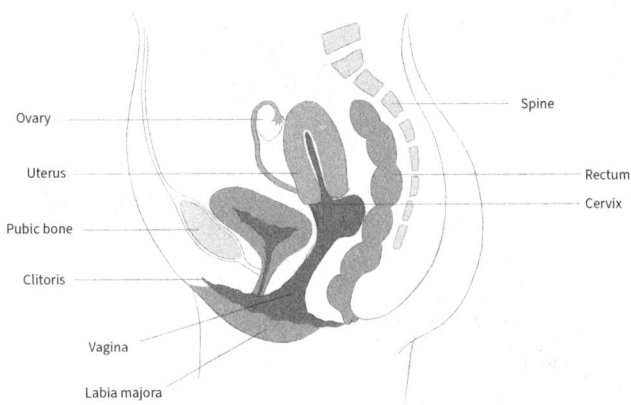

- *The inner and outer vaginal lips open.*

- *The outer third of the vagina becomes engorged and distended—the "orgasmic platform."*

- *The uterus is fully ascended.*

- *The end of the vagina is widely ballooned.*

- *The clitoris retracts under the clitoral hood.*

- *The tissues around the nipples fill with fluid, causing an apparent loss of nipple erection.*

As a woman, you don't have to be at this end point to be lubricated enough to enjoy penetrative sex, but that is the moment when you can experience the fullest sense of release and satisfaction.

In the orgasmic phase:

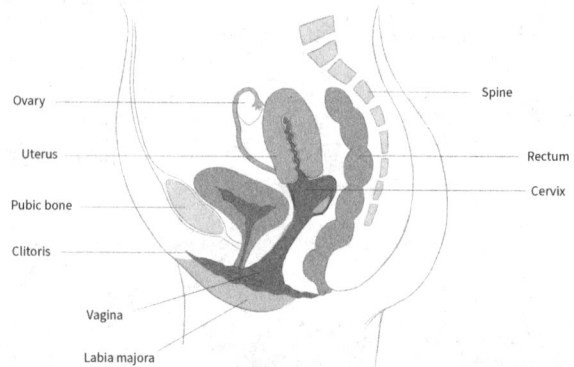

- *Most onscreen sex shows the woman having an orgasm via penetration with little foreplay. This would be exceedingly rare to the point I would question its existence.*

- *There are two types of female orgasm: external and internal, and they are linked.*

- *The external (clitoral) orgasm is more common and can happen during foreplay. It is unlikely to happen during penetration unless there is self-pleasuring or clitoral friction. Finger penetration is not the place to start; it will do nothing unless the internal clit is activated.*

- *The internal orgasm is linked to the external; the clitoris withdraws under the hood, the internal clitoris is activated, and at that point, the woman is ready for penetration and the internal orgasm becomes possible.*

- *Many women do not reach their orgasmic potential because of erection-led sex. However, this does not also mean they do not enjoy sex that is emotionally connected. Most women rated sex that had emotional satisfaction higher than sex with physical satisfaction.*

- *Physically, the breathing, heart rate, and blood pressure increase.*

- *Most body muscles tense.*

- *The uterus contracts.*

- *Pelvic floor muscles contract.*

- *The orgasmic platform pulsates.*

- *Contractions begin at 0.8-second intervals and recur 3 to 15 times.*

In the resolution phase:

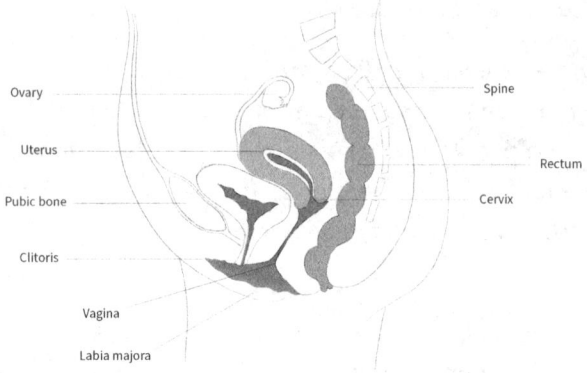

Ovary

Spine

Uterus

Rectum

Pubic bone

Cervix

Clitoris

Vagina

Labia majora

- *Breathing, heart rate, and blood pressure return to normal and muscles relax.*

- *Sex flush and swelling around nipples disappears.*

- *Clitoris returns to normal and the labia return to their unstimulated size.*

- *Orgasmic platform congestion disappears, and the uterus descends.*

- *The cervix remains open for 20 to 30 minutes, dipping into the seminal pool.*

- *Continued stimulation may produce further orgasms of varying intensity, as women have no refractory period.*

It is empowering and exciting to see the diagrams and understand how the uterus moves and lifts, opening the walls of the vagina, and how the clitoris (both external and internal) plays such a fundamental role in the phases of our sexual excitement through to orgasm. To have this knowledge to share with our partner in bringing awareness to our sexual play allows us to engage with the normality of the timing of our libidos and this understanding enables us to have more fulfilling sexual encounters.

While learning about the anatomy of arousal is important for all of us, and for intimacy practitioners it can bring a richer sense of authenticity to the scenes they create, it is just as valuable to understand the anatomy of sexual dysfunction. The reality is that 30–40 percent of people, men and women alike, will experience some form of sexual difficulty at some point in their lives. Knowing this not only helps us approach the subject with empathy, but also reminds us that these experiences are far more common than we might think. Some conditions of female sexual dysfunction include vaginismus, where the vaginal muscles involuntarily contract, making penetration, such as during intercourse or tampon insertion, painful or impossible; dyspareunia, which refers to difficult or painful sexual intercourse; and anorgasmia, the inability to reach orgasm (a condition that can affect both men and women). In men, sexual dysfunction can include erectile dysfunction, premature ejaculation, and delayed ejaculation.

This was brilliantly highlighted in *Men Up,* the second program I worked on with Russell T Davies that told the story of a trial for Viagra that took place in Wales in 1984. Beautifully written by Matthew Barry, it showed the importance of men talking about their fears and concerns. By finding a sense of camaraderie with each other, and exploring erectile dysfunction in open and honest ways, they managed to enrich their relationships. Men watching the program responded to the way it opened up topics that they found difficult to talk about.[5] Likewise, in

Sex Education, the condition of vaginismus was beautifully explored through the character of Lily, played by Tanya Reynolds, where "Fans of the show are calling its portrayal of vaginismus groundbreaking—especially because it shows that the condition doesn't have to mean the end of sexual pleasure."[6]

I firmly believe that the detail of both men's and women's anatomy of arousal and dysfunction should be part of our sex education, shared at an age-appropriate point in school, as part of active consent and positive sex education. I will discuss this in the next chapter.

Blair goes on to say the following:

- *Good sex involves curiosity, which often involves some speaking and negotiation; without this, we are all fumbling in the dark.*
- *Self-pleasuring is often a necessary part of sex; it helps to show your partner what you like as well as getting you higher on the ladder.*
- *Use of fantasy in long-term relationships is important. This can come from others or from each other.*
- *Toys can be important too. For older couples, who might have less sensitivity, toys are an essential part of pleasure. Vibrating bullets, for example, can help intensify the experience for both men and women. Some women cannot get to orgasm without a toy, and that's OK. It's important to de-shame this and for society to stop believing that toys are for kinks and hen parties.*

All of this is not much understood and certainly not much talked about on film or anywhere else. The length of the female cycle of arousal accounts for a woman's ability to break off from intimacy to answer the door, or to attend to a crying child or a ringing telephone. It takes a longer amount of time for a woman to be fully aroused and engaged in an intimate act, whereas a male cycle of desire is far more goal-focused. Men feel desire and they head more directly for orgasm. However, in long-term relationships, often where children are involved, men will also often initiate intimacy from a position of neutrality rather than spontaneous arousal.

To put it more simply, desire, which we see onscreen as coming first, will sometimes, and very often, come last. Blair puts it this way: in long-term domestic relationships in the real world, you could have sex, but you could also do the washing up. Intimate activity is assessed; it is not, in a domestic setting, necessarily more important than anything else. When you are in that place, the appropriate stimuli for intimate engagement will be entirely different—and those stimuli will have to take account of all the little inconveniences of life together. For example, in the morning, one partner might wake up feeling ready for sex, and the other might say, "Oh, go and brush your teeth first." That doesn't mean that intimacy or even sexual relations can't take place. It just means the starting point is different.

In her work as a sexual therapist, Blair meets couples who fear that the fact that it takes a woman so much longer to get into sex than her partner means she has low libido. As shown, this is not the case—it is just that their libido is different. The sex scenes that show women immediately responding to physical touch and always being turned on within a few minutes of kissing are simply unrealistic.

So is the everlasting erection perpetuated by pornography, yet often depicted in mainstream films as well. What men tend to see onscreen is an erection that arrives extremely fast, without stimulation, and then just stays until penetration. If men can't achieve this in the bedroom, they worry there is something wrong with them and go to the doctor concerned they have erectile dysfunction. The truth is that most men, especially if they are over 20, don't have spontaneous erections without being touched—and all erections naturally go up and down during intercourse.

It is, for example, normal for there to be no erection if the man is pleasuring his partner—or when he is reaching for lubrication or a condom. It doesn't mean the man isn't experiencing enjoyment (the erection isn't always the only sign of psychological arousal), and it is likely that the erection will return after genital stimulation and toward the point of penetration. I am not suggesting that we have to see all of this onscreen all the time. But as creative filmmakers, the suggestion of some of these realities would save a lot of suffering in the real world.

The prevalence of pornography is leading to other, more dangerous myths. In pornography, the scenes people are watching tend to last about 20 minutes. This can make men worry about the time between penetration and ejaculation. They think they are suffering from premature ejaculation if they only last 15 minutes. Yet the completely normal time between penetration and ejaculation is somewhere around 5 to 7 minutes. Medically premature ejaculation is defined as under a minute.[7]

This isn't the only way sexually explicit videos distort attitudes to intercourse and intimacy. If men watch the entire 20-minute pornography short while masturbating, then they are creating delayed ejaculation. In heterosexual couples, this creates female disorders because women are not able to be penetrated for that long without getting sore and dry. They arrive at the doctor or the therapist worrying about sexual pain, but it is often uncomfortable for women to be penetrated for so long. The increased prescription of Viagra for older men has compounded this problem in older couples. When people brag about having had sex all night long, it really isn't something to aim for.

At the moment, we seem to be trapped in a cycle of sexual dysfunction: men watch pornography and think it is what women want. Which it isn't! Then they think they are doing something wrong—yet it is what they are seeing that is unreal, not what they are doing. This might explain the rise in reports of men trying to strangle women during sex, another pornographic trope and not often something women want except within very careful and preset parameters. Erotic asphyxiation has been practiced in BDSM communities for centuries, but it has historically involved doing it to oneself. What is new is the rise in sexual strangulation and the way it is widely perceived as normal, with little or no awareness of its potential health consequences.

In July 2024, researchers from Melbourne and Queensland Universities in Australia published a study that showed that over half of the 4,702 people aged between 18 and 35 years old who had been questioned had choked or been choked by a sexual partner.[8] Fifty-seven percent had been strangled during sex at least once, and 51 percent had choked a partner at least once. The first time in both cases was usually between the ages of

19 and 21. More women (61 percent) than men (43 percent) reported having been choked at least once, with more men (59 percent) than women (40 percent) saying they had choked their partners. For trans and gender-diverse people, the rates were higher still, with 78 percent reporting that they had been choked and 74 percent reporting that they had choked their partners.

People said they found out about sexual choking through various sources, most commonly pornography (61 percent) but also through films (40 percent), friends (32 percent), social media (31 percent), and discussions with current or potential partners (29 percent).[9]

For some people, sexual asphyxiation is an exciting part of sex play and games that they enjoy. Even then, it is really concerning that in the pursuit of erotic pleasure, people are willing to risk brain damage and, in extreme cases, death. Sexual choking is dangerous physically, mentally, and emotionally, and so the fact that young people seem to regard it as part of normal intimate activity is alarming. If they don't know what they are doing, and what they are risking, then the dangers are greater.

A similar concern has also arisen around the rise in anal sex among heterosexual couples. The gay community has long experience of sexual penetration in this way and understands the need both for anal hygiene and for lubrication. As the practice has become more common between heterosexual couples, many women are suffering anal tearing and severe discomfort.

In life, as on film, the definitions of sex can be expanded. Not everything has to be focused around penetration, which can become painful, particularly in older women, where the vaginal walls are thinner. It's important, I think, for us all to recognize that sex isn't just an act; it's an experience. A massage between two people might be a gesture of intimacy, and self-pleasure in harmony might be more satisfying and bonding than a penetrative act that might be uncomfortable for one party.

Penetration isn't even necessarily the most intimate part of sexual intercourse, yet couples rush to it because they are perhaps wary of the greater intimacy and exposure that nonpenetrative sex requires. Mutual pleasuring, touching, and massage are in some ways more revealing than simply moving toward penetrative intercourse; they take more time. It might be possible to find greater happiness by exploring more. We need to expand the script, both on- and offscreen.

There's one thing that would begin to solve all of these difficulties in intimate relationships, and that's the simplest thing in the world. We need to talk more. As Linsey Blair told me: "Somehow, it's seen as unsexy to talk during sex. But one of the biggest myths of all is that somehow, as if by magic, we know what our partner is thinking, and we can communicate our desires without speech. For normal people, in normal relationships, it's really useful to talk. You need to be able to say, 'I'm not sure I want to do that,' or, 'I'm not comfortable with that,' or alternatively, 'I really like that,' or, 'That feels great. Keep doing that.' Just by telling each other what they want, couples can change what they are doing, and that's essential to sex and consent."

In our own intimate lives, we cannot assume we know what is going on inside our partner's head. Nor can we assume that because they seemed to like something last time, or they consented to a particular sexual movement, that they are going to want it again. Active consent never ends, and talking is an essential part of it. It isn't unsexy to talk; in fact, it can often lead to greater sexual fulfillment and deeper, more satisfying intimate relationships.

Blair points out that male gay sex tends to have much more negotiation in it than straight sex because penetration is not necessarily a guarantee and who is going to be penetrated needs consideration. With female gay intimacy, there tends to be more negotiation than in straight sex, but less than in male gay sex.

I think it's true to say that talking and negotiation are nearly always missing from the sex we see onscreen. What is presented as sexy all too often is the man taking over the sex and being quite dominant and a woman being responsive. What we hardly ever see is sex going wrong. Yet we can learn the most when we try something and it's a disaster. Blair told me about one couple she had been helping where she'd suggested a particular exercise, and the woman had returned the following week saying it had been terrible. Her husband had touched her breasts, and she had begun to cry, so they stopped having sex and hugged.

Blair could reassure her that it wasn't a disaster. It was an intimate moment. Loving one another, hugging, reassuring each other are all parts of intimacy. If we can talk about something that has gone wrong, it creates an emotional connection that is probably the most important part of an intimate relationship. Our definitions need to expand to take account of this.

Blair's account made me think of *Men Up,* which showed couples struggling in their relationships and resolving difficulties through talking and understanding.

For example, one plot line showed a woman who has a double mastectomy around the same time as her husband gradually becomes impotent. She is trying to find a way back to an acceptance of her body, while he is worrying that he can't have an erection. After he takes the Viagra, they do have sex, and it is uncomfortable for her—while he is desperate to have intercourse through to orgasm. It's really not good sex—and the scene shows that, which is brilliant. Because then, on another occasion, something happens that turns both of them on, and they go upstairs and have sex again. She is more empowered, and he touches her, telling her how beautiful she is. They connect intimately, lovingly. There's a progression, and what we are seeing onscreen is helpful as well as telling an absorbing story.

I'm not saying that all this talking is easy. Most people find it difficult and embarrassing to discuss their sexual and intimate needs. I'm a fan of *The Good Sex Project* podcast made in New Zealand by Melody Thomas, who talks to real-life couples and experts about their sexual and romantic lives.[10] Episode 4 in series 1 is called "What Are You Into?," which is a great place to start when wanting to open out a conversation with a partner. The fundamental advice for clear communication is the same as that in the Intimacy on Set Guidelines: it's important to be open, honest, and as straightforward as you can be.

You might want to discuss contraception, the kind of foreplay that turns you on, the areas of your body that are most responsive to touch and stimulation. As you talk, you might decide to share sexual fantasies or to share a desire for sex toys.

As you move into a sexual encounter, it's also important to remember that consent is an ongoing process—and so is communication. Sometimes this will be verbal—encouraging activities that feel good, and gently discouraging things you don't like. But some communication is also nonverbal; you can shift position or move your partner's hand to make it clear what turns you on.

Terrence Real, a family therapist and author, argued in an article that couples having these kinds of debates and discussions, even having rows, is not a bad thing. "Our culture worships the harmony phase, but a good relationship thrives on surviving the mess. The work of intimacy is the collision of imperfections and how we manage those."[11] I absolutely agree with that. In my ideal world, we need much more of this kind of understanding; a realization that all relationships aren't simply happy or sad, but most are somewhere in the middle. They don't develop in straight lines. They are about closeness, which gets reduced or disrupted; in happy relationships, they return to closeness. They are messy, imperfect things that require work, not to be covered in a Hollywood happy ending.

Sex scenes that enhance our understanding of intimacy can linger in the imagination for all the right reasons. The most famous, and in many people's view the most successful, scene of film lovemaking is the one between Julie Christie and Donald Sutherland in *Don't Look Now*, directed by Nicolas Roeg.

Roeg and Christie had already worked together many times; you feel the trust between the actors and the director. It shows a married couple living through the tragic death of their daughter, all their emotions raw, making love on a holiday to Venice. It still looks real in a way that very few scenes of intimacy do, so truthful in fact that it has persistently led to stories that Christie and Sutherland were actually making love. Yet according to Sutherland, it was performed to the sound of a very loud Arriflex camera— "like a Singer sewing machine on methamphetamines"— and the choreography was entirely of the "put your hand there" variety.[12]

But in editing the scenes of the couple's lovemaking with quiet images of them calmly getting dressed for dinner, the genius of Roeg and editor Graeme Clifford transformed it into something very special, a scene that people relate to and remember with pleasure. It has a languid quality, unfolding with time. It tells the story of a married couple rediscovering their love for each other in the shadow of tragedy; it is integral to the plot, not gratuitous. It is a scene about love and life, about true intimacy.[13] When you see something like that, you feel the power of scenes that increase our understanding of what it is to be intimate.

It is also important to change the gaze of what we see so that it does not encompass just the male or female point of view but also every community. Scenes of LGBTQ+ intimacy are more accepted onscreen, thanks to the pioneering work of series such as *Gentleman Jack* and *It's a Sin* and films such as *Portrait of a Lady on Fire*. However, scenes depicting trans intimacy are still rare. So are stories where one or both of the characters are disabled, though I am proud of the work we did on *Ralph & Katie* by Peter Bowker, which showed two people with Down syndrome having a loving relationship as a couple. By honoring everybody's diversity and showing those relationships onscreen, in all their richness, we expand the definition of intimate relationships and varied bodies in ordinary life.

This matters. I worked with one actor who, like 1 to 5 percent of the population, had a third nipple. When I checked in about their requirements about being fully naked, they had only one: that on no account was their third nipple to be covered by makeup or tape. They told me that in the past, when they had acted in scenes with a bare chest, people had contacted them to say thank you, because they had made having a third nipple as natural and normal as it is. In showing it, they were helping others.

In our conversations about intimacy, Dr. Orna Guralnik has pointed out that she believes that the truth and dignity about the filming of intimacy that intimacy practitioners are bringing behind the scenes has an effect on what the viewer sees. The Intimacy on Set Guidelines put in place a professional process and a structure that makes it really clear that the actors are simulating a sexual act as a character, not becoming involved in it as people. We take care of them personally so that artistically and professionally they can step into the character and the story.

With simulated scenes of intimacy, actors have barriers, cushions, flesh-colored garments, and so on in place, so they can be as protected as they want to be. But because they feel safe and happy, they can fill themselves with the detail of character and story and step into the narrative. Precisely because they can do that, they can tell stories that are revealing about intimacy and the vulnerabilities it causes without themselves being personally vulnerable.

For Dr. Guralnik, this sets up a virtuous feedback loop.

Because the frame they are working within is so safe, it makes intimate scenes more powerful and more truthful. This is what she said to me: "It's like the difference between locker room and bro talk and conversations that treat sex with dignity and respect. If you are helping actors approach their intimate moments with a different paradigm in mind, that's what they convey when they are acting. They are, by way of mirror neurons, conveying to the public a different approach to sexuality, gender relations, and sexual politics.

"This can have a profound effect on what in psycho-analytic jargon we call the imaginary—which is what people imagine before they do it. The way they represent life to themselves internally. In that sense I think the intimacy work you are doing is huge. It's not just affecting the experience of writers and directors, but it's also projected into the psyche of the viewer, the witness if you like, morphing that psyche from within by way of identification. The care with which the actors and the subject matter is handled registers with the viewer not only in a linear, explicit way but implicitly, by a kind of osmosis. You are introducing a deep change in ethics."

It's a question of dreaming into and imagining what you want happening. I found that increasing my understanding of the difference between male and female sexual arousal in my work with Linsey Blair vastly deepened my own recognition of my normal, and what I could expect and what I wanted. That consideration of my needs and sharing them with my partner—and encouraging him to do the same—was a positive thing to take into my intimate life. That's the paradigm shift in the real world.

If something isn't quite working for you, you can explore

that, seeking out books or websites I recommend on pages 345–53 or just having conversations with friends. When you understand yourself in a new way, you can bring something fresh and present it to your partner, always being mindful of asking your partner what they want. The care with which we handle our own relationships can also bring about change, so that in our own lives too, we can create a better frame in which to have more powerful intimate encounters.

CHAPTER NINE

SEX EDUCATION

I remember my sex education vividly. We did a bit in biology lessons about the basic anatomy of male and female genitalia which, since I attended a Catholic girls' day school, was just about as basic as it was possible to be. I can see our poor biology teacher to this day, some 45 years later. She was at that point about eight and a half months pregnant, and she stood with her hands behind her back, leaning against a wall, eyes fixed firmly on the floor, going more and more pink as she spoke. "Sexual intercourse," she said firmly, "only happens inside the bounds of matrimony. And only to a loving couple, with the intention of having a baby."

That was absolutely it. Nothing about contraception, protection, or consent. Nothing about how sex actually worked. When I met my first boyfriend, at the age of 18, I literally didn't have a clue about anything. I knew nothing about the logistics of sex and intimacy. I was completely unprepared. As for the idea that sex might be pleasurable, that was never spoken about.

Things have changed since then, thank goodness, but it is true to say that in the 2020s, the way we talk about sex to our teenagers is still sadly lacking, often leaving them in a state of unhappiness and confusion. It is still true in a lot of cases that in sex education, the way we talk about intercourse is essentially sex prevention. It is all about anticipating what might go wrong—the unwanted pregnancies and the sexually transmitted diseases (STDs). If you are lucky enough to have any discussion about sex in your school, then all too often it is only about putting a condom on correctly. One of the most hilariously truthful scenes in the first season of *Sex Education* is when—after an outbreak of pubic lice—the biology teacher is reluctantly coerced into taking a class where Otis and Maeve have to practice putting a condom on a plastic erect penis. Cue embarrassment and much hilarity.

Although exaggerated, that really wasn't far from the truth. Certainly, while my own children's conversations about sex in school were a whole lot better than my convent school experience, their education still did not equip them with a positive understanding of their sexual awakening. They were taught how not to have sex because of the lurking dangers, and how to use contraception. Quite often, the information came tinged with the same semi-Christian morality that colored my own upbringing.

The difficulty with this approach is that teenagers do have sex, and if your only strategy is to try to stop them, then it is doomed to failure. What's more, teenagers are now utterly surrounded by images of sex and sexualized behavior online. If I have been generally worried as I outlined in the last chapter about the way that pornographic tropes have become mainstream, my concern is greater when it comes to children and teenagers. Not a day goes by without some news story about the unregulated spread of pornography and sexualized images on social media leading children into darker and darker territory. I've heard stories about 9-year-olds who have watched pornography without having the first understanding of how their bodies work or what they are watching. At the time of writing this book, there were reports of girls aged 14 and 15 turning up at school with strangulation marks on their necks because their boyfriends had watched pornographic videos and thought that was how sex was done. As I've said before, what we see onscreen can become our main form of education when education elsewhere is lacking. A report by the Children's Commissioner for England, Dame Rachel de Souza, in January 2023, discovered that 1 in 10 children had watched pornography by the time they were 9 and that a quarter of pupils in their final year of primary school (aged 11) had already been exposed to it. Four out of five (79 percent) had seen pornography involving violence by the time they were 18.[1] In the US, one study found 42 percent of young people between the ages of 10 and 17 reported viewing online pornography. Other studies showed that 19 to 37 percent of teenagers reported intentional use, while unintentional pornography use in adolescents ranged from 35 percent to 66 percent.[2]

De Souza described pornography's harmful effects. Nearly half of the 16- to 21-year-olds who took part in the survey assumed girls either "expect" or "enjoy" sex that involves physical aggression such as airway restriction. One girl described her first kiss with a boy aged 12 who tried to strangle her; he thought it was normal. Faced with the danger of encountering such practices, some girls are— understandably—swearing off sexual encounters all together. In this way, children are being sexualized before they've ever had a girlfriend or a boyfriend, before they've kissed or held hands, before they've begun to explore one another's bodies. Their sexual discovery is out of kilter with their own experience; they are seeing pictures of intercourse before they have even held hands. As they grow older, this disconnect between their lived experience of their sexuality and what they believe they should be experiencing deepens. As I explore later in this chapter, what they are seeing and what they believe others are doing can condition their own behavior, leading to anxiety (why aren't I behaving like my peers?) and abuse as they copy what they think others are doing.

The Everyone's Invited website was set up in the UK in June 2020 by Soma Sara after she watched *I May Destroy You*. In allowing survivors of rape culture to share their anonymous testimonies, it uncovered a hidden world of abuse in schools and universities, where—in Sara's words—attitudes, behaviors, and beliefs in society have the effect of normalizing and trivializing sexual violence. She defines rape culture as including misogyny, rape jokes, sexual harassment, online sexual abuse (upskirting, nonconsensual sharing of intimate photos, cyberflashing), and sexual coercion. The survivors' horrifying testimonies included examples of sexual assault and rape. The group is now working in schools with an education program designed to promote healthy relationships and sexual well-being.

I first started to think deeply about the way our young people learn about intimacy when I realized that the Intimacy on Set Guidelines needed to be extended to the way drama was being taught in schools. If young people are doing high school drama, taking advanced theater courses, or studying performing arts through technical programs, then it seems important to me that the guidelines that protect them are followed. I'd heard many stories of, for example, geography or PE teachers leading drama classes and proceeding without any guidance about what to do. They might be studying *Romeo and Juliet* and encouraging their two teenage leads to kiss; if you're performing at the age of 14, that might be your first experience of a kiss, and it's happening in the full view of your classmates who are egging you on.

In one example, a 13-year-old girl, who had been cast as Liesl in a school production of *The Sound of Music,* was told by her director to kiss the boy playing Rolf. He was 18, and therefore technically an adult. It was entirely inappropriate that a director should be telling the boy to put his hands all over a prepubescent girl. Fortunately, he had the sense to say no, as he didn't feel that was right. But there wasn't a framework in place where both parties could set their boundaries and agree how they were going to work. In this context, I wanted to encourage schools to use the Intimacy on Set Guidelines just as much as university drama courses and professional bodies. But at the same time, I realized that it would be difficult to do this unless the institutions were already working from a bedrock of agreement and consent, equipping their pupils to have the language to call their boundaries, as well as a having a fully integrated and positive sexual education program.

Around that time, a colleague introduced me to Dr. Siobhán O'Higgins, who has been promoting sexual health since the 1990s and who now works from the Department of Psychology at Galway University in Ireland. Her PhD in 2011 explored what young Irish people want to learn and how they wanted to be talked to about sexuality and relationships. Building on that, Dr. O'Higgins has worked extensively in schools, with children, teenagers and young people and with teachers and parents, developing better ways of educating youngsters about sexuality and relationships.

Dr. O'Higgins is one of the leads on the Active* Consent program. The data from Active* Consent's research is the basis for the development of workshops, dramas, and training that all aim to empower teenagers by raising awareness of the importance of communication and sharing ideas, from other young people, about what one could actually say, all based on an understanding that consent needs to be OMFG—Ongoing, Mutual, and Freely Given. The organization's ConsentHub states their aim as: "The Active* Consent program believes that the most effective form of consent education supports teenagers' sexual health and agency and is taught through a sex positive lens which honors people's choices whether or not they choose to become sexually active."[3]

Dr. O'Higgins and I have worked together closely, developing sessions to be delivered in secondary schools, to pupils, parents, and teachers, using scenes from productions I have worked on to offer examples of active consent in action. This forms the groundwork to then share the process and ethos of the Intimacy on Set Guidelines with teachers, parents, and students engaged in drama, be it the General Certificate of Secondary Education (GCSE) and A-level curriculum or in drama clubs.

One of the most fascinating aspects of Active* Consent's research is the way it reveals a social norm gap between how important teenagers think things are and how comfortable they are around issues of sexuality and what they think their peers are thinking and doing.

In a seminar with teenagers aged 17 (which is the Irish age of consent), Dr. O'Higgins asked whether it was important to have consent before engaging in any kind of sexual activity including fingering, blow jobs, and so on. A majority, 93 percent of females and 79 percent of males, agreed that it was. However, when the teenagers were asked whether their peers and other people their age thought consent before sexual activity was important, only 54 percent of females and 50 percent of males believed others agreed with them. This is an extraordinary gap between reality and perception. It creates individualized peer pressure because teenagers genuinely think consent is important—but do not believe that other people think it is important. What stops the majority asking for consent, or conforming to a kind of behavior they know in their hearts is correct, is the incorrect belief that others don't agree.

Teenagers don't want to stand out. They want to find their own tribe in order to reduce their own vulnerability. Yet this misconception gap pushes them into behavior they are not comfortable with. The barriers to communicating consent range from feeling pressured and afraid to ask for consent to not knowing how to bring in consent when caught up in the moment. Teenagers feel "afraid" of rejection, of being judged, of disappointing or offending or ruining the mood. What helps consent and communication is awareness and education; talking to others opens out the conversation and gives confidence. Having the opportunity to role play and try out the ways in which they can both ask for consent that does not ruin the mood, as well as to be able to pause if something is happening that is beyond what they are comfortable with, and to have the language to be able to invite consent, to slow things down, keeps them feeling comfortable and respected.

The data goes on to reveal that if teenagers are asked about their own levels of comfort with different kinds of intimacy, only 7 percent of girls feel comfortable with someone touching them under their clothes. Yet they believe 43 percent of their peers would be comfortable with doing that, for example.

With boys, the statistics reveal that just over 30 percent would be comfortable having oral sex or sexual intercourse with someone they have just met, so a majority—the remaining 70 percent—would not. This cuts against the gender sexual stereotype that boys are always up for instant sexual contact. That idea is perpetuated by sexualized social media—not just by the easily accessible and omnipresent porn sites but by the sexual messages young people receive through all forms of online interaction.

"If you actually show them the data, they recognize that everybody is just like them," says Dr. O'Higgins. "They realize that they are not just an insecure little person who doesn't know. Everybody doesn't know. They are all amateurs when it comes to sexual encounters. That is why this work is so important. In workshops and drama shows and films we can show them a different, more truthful script." This is beautifully depicted by Hazel Mead in the *Sex Education We Wish We'd Had* illustration that Active* Consent included in their presentations to teenagers.

All of these issues were clearly dramatized in Molly Manning Walker's remarkable film *How to Have Sex,*

THE SEX EDUCATION WE WISH WE'D HAD

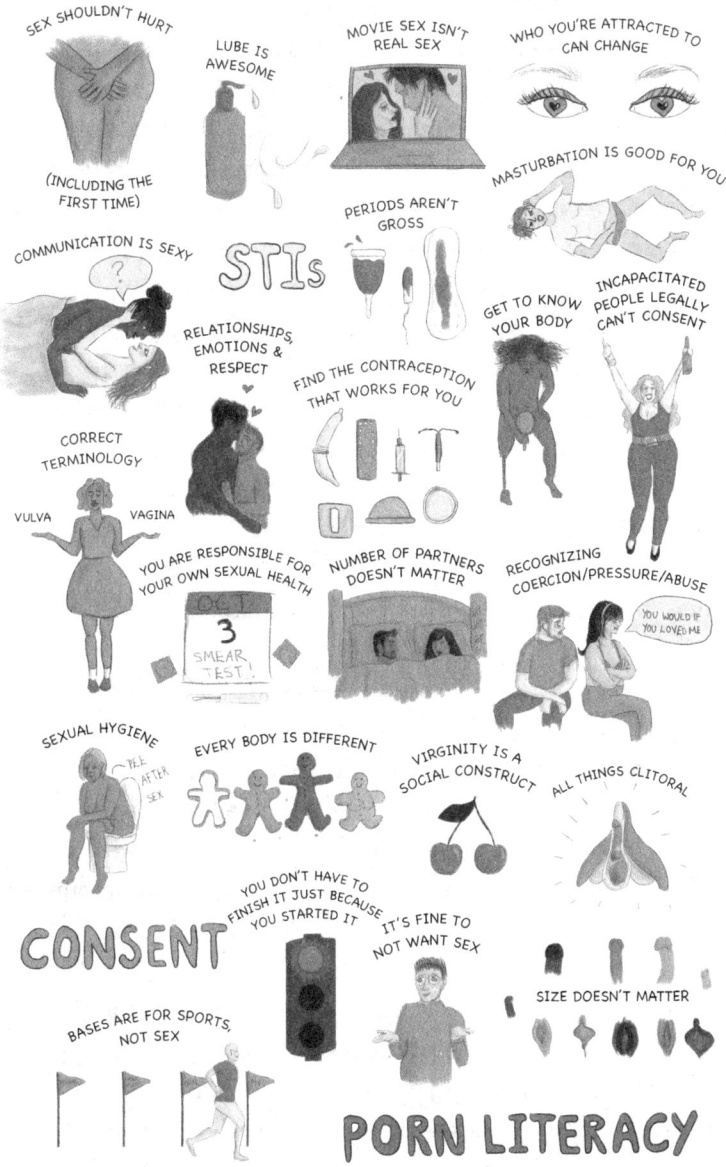

released in 2023. The British director turned her camera on a group of post-GCSE girls hell-bent on partying in Crete and produced a searing study of consent that poses uncomfortable questions about consent and the coercive influence of peers. The film is brilliant and vibrant but also almost unbearable to watch, truly heartbreaking in the level of misunderstanding it reveals.

The misconception gap Dr. O'Higgins talks about leads the girls into behavior they are not comfortable with, as depicted in the character of 16-year-old Tara (brilliantly played by Mia McKenna-Bruce), who is pushed by her friend Skye to lose her virginity during the alcohol- and party-fueled holiday. Tara meets one boy, Badger (Shaun Thomas), who she likes and who is kind to her. But circumstances and their inability to talk to one another keep pushing them apart, and Tara ends up being manipulated and coerced into an abusive sexual encounter with another boy.

The way that scene develops—a rape in all but name—is devastating. As the critic Wendy Ide remarks: "Tara's increasing discomfort with the way the holiday plays out and the sex that eventually happens is revealed not so much in dialogue—the whole point of the film is that she, and girls her age, lack the crucial vocabulary to talk about their needs and experiences—but in McKenna-Bruce's mercurially expressive face."[4]

The scenes of assault were clearly choreographed by Manning Walker and the production's intimacy coordinator. The first scene convincingly tracks Tara's unease as she's coaxed to get into the sea by the apparently charming Paddy (played by Samuel Bottomley)—and then told to take her clothes off, and then forced into sex. At each point, he overrides her protests, and her unhappiness and her inability to get him to stop are upsetting to watch. So are the scenes afterward, where her friends tease her about the encounter, never for a moment spotting the trauma it has caused her. There is also a later encounter, when he again assaults her as she is lying on a bed and she tries even harder to get him to stop. Throughout, he never registers he is doing anything wrong.

As writer and director Manning Walker fed her own experiences into the story and as part of the preproduction process, the filmmakers held focus groups with young people. They encountered girls who suggested that they could only protect themselves by wearing more clothes and drinking less. These interviews convinced Manning Walker of the importance of making the film. As her star McKenna-Bruce noted in an interview: "Somewhere along the way, the lines have been blurred. Sex is between two humans and where have we lost that humanity?"[5]

The film has inspired conversations that have continued. When I met Manning Walker at a screening, she told me she was going into schools with The Schools Consent Project, a company that aims to "normalize conversations about consent in order to safeguard young people and drive down sexual offending rates."[6] Some boys they met felt the behavior depicted in the sexual encounters between Paddy and Tara were OK; they couldn't see what was wrong with his behavior. Yet in the class, other boys explained to them why it wasn't right and talked about issues of consent.

What all this makes clear is that in supporting our teenagers, encouraging them not only to listen to the wisdom they have inside that allows them to recognize and call out the gray areas of consent but also to have the language to call a halt to any sexual behavior that is overstepping their boundaries, they can learn to be empowered people who develop respect both for themselves and for others. When we highlight to our teenagers, particularly our young boys and men, the difference between coercion—which is about power—and intimacy, connection, and love, which comes with consent, they can make considered choices that nurture relationships and human connection. Acting out hypothetical situations can help our teenagers understand consent.

Watching a scenario play out makes things clear. If they hear someone saying stop, see the nonverbal signals, and experience how to read both the verbal and physical signals when a person is not exactly saying no but is certainly not giving free consent, it will help them in their own intimate lives. If this education is happening in secondary school, to equip them with a sense of self, boundaries, and consent before they finish their GCSE year, they will have the equipment to make informed decisions to navigate their social life with confidence and respect for themselves and their peers. However, for our children to grow up with their sense of self intact, this awareness and focus would benefit from starting right from primary and junior school, which we shall come to later in the chapter.

Programs such as The Schools Consent Project, Everyone's Invited, and Active* Consent are going some way to provide this positive education in our schools. However, for fundamental change to be embedded, the issue needs to be taken up by governments and implemented in an organized way. In Australia, where studies show that one in three Australian women have experienced physical and/or sexual violence perpetrated by a man since the age of 15, consent education became mandatory in 2023.[7] The curriculum includes holistic and age-appropriate consent education from kindergarten to year 10, with topics including information about power imbalances, gendered stereotypes, and coercion. It would be great if something similar could be adopted worldwide, beginning in primary schools.

Meanwhile, Active* Consent, and other organizations like them, are engaging with young people on TikTok and other social media, trying to balance the mass of misinformation about intimacy and sexual behavior that is out there. It is an uphill struggle because the misinformation isn't just coming from children and teenagers sharing misleading information about their own sexual activities—many teenagers are reluctant to admit that they are less experienced and less confident than they believe their peers to be—but also from other older influencers who deliberately manipulate the expectations of children and teenagers for their own purposes.

Dr. O'Higgins points out that the influence of Andrew Tate and other online influencers and podcasters is dangerous because young people expect adults to offer them sensible advice. In the early 2020s, Tate built up a huge online following among young men by promoting an extremely misogynistic position and suggesting that an ultramasculine lifestyle was a way to live. His suggestion was that to be happy you needed to be strong, to make money, and to have a lot of sex. He talked about hitting and choking women, trashing their belongings, and stopping them from going out.

Tate and his brother, Tristan, were charged in Romania

in December 2023 over allegations of rape, human trafficking, and forming an organized group to sexually exploit women, charges they denied. His TikTok account was taken down, yet before then, it had been watched more than 11.6 billion times.[8] A report in one British newspaper suggested that three-quarters of people viewing videos posted under the Tate hashtag in the UK were aged between 18 and 24.[9] The Center for Countering Digital Hate further suggested that children as young as 13 were being exposed to his videos.[10]

If you combine their susceptibility to such views with the fact that only 23 percent of youngsters in one Active* Consent survey thought that the sex education they were receiving in schools was adequate, then another information gap opens. It's clear that teenagers aren't receiving positive sex education that will support them in their sexual awakening and into their adult lives with a consent-driven view of intimacy.

The illustration by Hazel Mead on page 255 shows a list of all the things they wish were discussed in sex education: that communication is sexy, the realization that film sex isn't real sex, that periods aren't gross, that gender is theirs to decide, and that more porn literacy is needed. It also includes issues of body positivity: clear information about their bodies, and a recognition that every body is different. Another Hazel Mead image used by Dr. O'Higgins that I love shows the things you don't see in mainstream porn, such as period sex, safe words, running to get the toilet paper, pimply butts, laughter, and falling off the bed!

There is a general acceptance among educators that these are topics that should be covered—Dr. O'Higgins says she is always struck by how grateful teachers are for

THINGS YOU DON'T SEE IN MAINSTREAM PORN

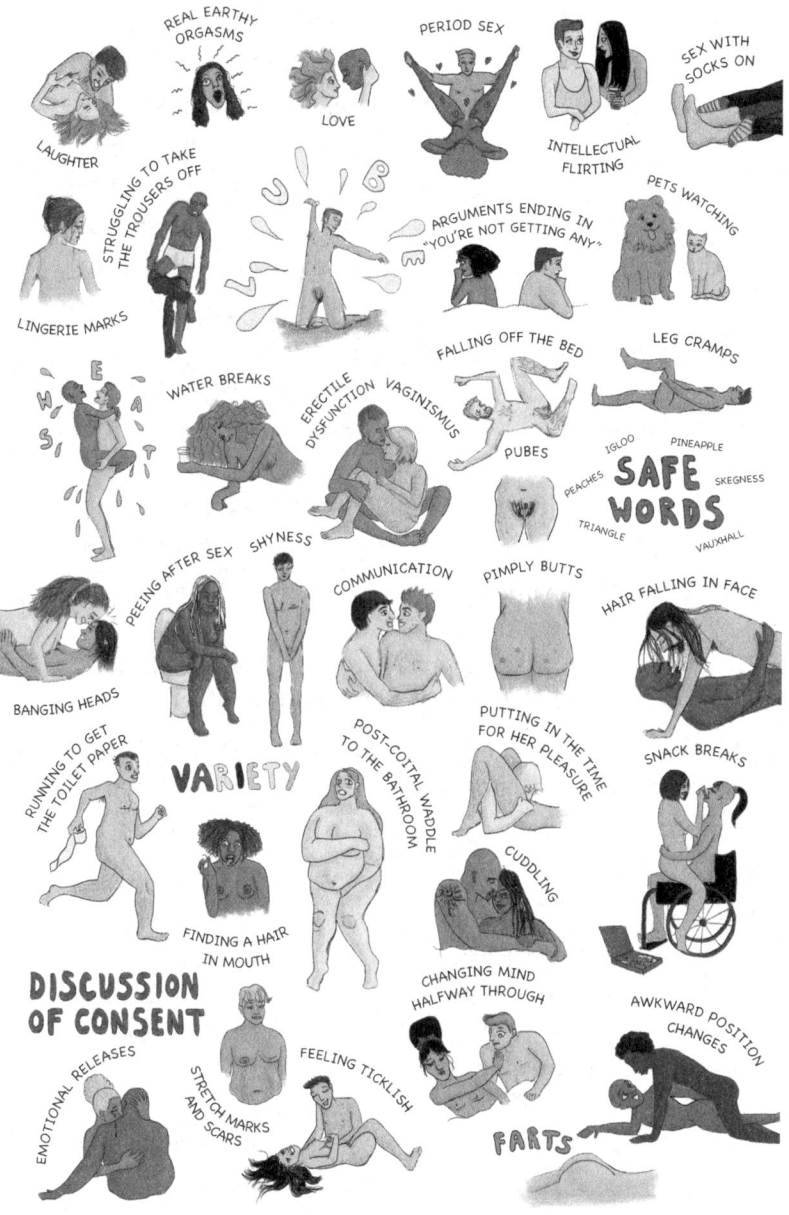

LAUGHTER

REAL EARTHY ORGASMS

LOVE

PERIOD SEX

INTELLECTUAL FLIRTING

SEX WITH SOCKS ON

STRUGGLING TO TAKE THE TROUSERS OFF

ARGUMENTS ENDING IN "YOU'RE NOT GETTING ANY"

PETS WATCHING

LINGERIE MARKS

WATER BREAKS

ERECTILE DYSFUNCTION

VAGINISMUS

FALLING OFF THE BED

LEG CRAMPS

PUBES

SAFE WORDS

IGLOO PINEAPPLE

PEACHES SKEGNESS

TRIANGLE VAUXHALL

PEEING AFTER SEX

SHYNESS

COMMUNICATION

PIMPLY BUTTS

HAIR FALLING IN FACE

BANGING HEADS

RUNNING TO GET THE TOILET PAPER

VARIETY

POST-COITAL WADDLE TO THE BATHROOM

PUTTING IN THE TIME FOR HER PLEASURE

CUDDLING

SNACK BREAKS

FINDING A HAIR IN MOUTH

CHANGING MIND HALFWAY THROUGH

AWKWARD POSITION CHANGES

DISCUSSION OF CONSENT

EMOTIONAL RELEASES

STRETCH MARKS AND SCARS

FEELING TICKLISH

FARTS

261

the workshops that she runs. Many teachers said things such as, "I really just wanted to get involved in giving them the correct, positive information," "I think they need to know but they might not understand what they need to know. There's like a gap in their mind, like, you know, for example they might hear the word consent, but the gap is there, what does that really mean. It's kind of like filling in the blanks," and, "All the teachers . . . found it really profound and, you know, so relevant to what's going on."

But there are still many hurdles to be overcome in our intention to deliver better conversations about intimacy to help our teenagers and young people to be safer and more confident. As Dr. O'Higgins points out, if we can get the balance right, then we are actually helping teenagers and young people to preserve their innocence rather than lose it. If they understand that the images that are all around them are not necessarily a truthful depiction of sexual activity, then it will be easier for them to find their own way to having satisfying and safe sexual encounters that conform with what they want, rather than with anyone else's expectations.

It is important to strike the right tone in these conversations. Dr. O'Higgins explains that in the sessions she runs, she often uses humor to overcome the embarrassment and giggles that so often interrupt Personal, Social, Health and Economic education (PSHE) sessions as children get to grips with their own changing bodies, flooded with hormones and new feelings. At primary level, they will find it hilarious that they have dangly bits and that things stick up and smell. If you can pitch conversations at a level where they are comfortable, then it helps them to explore their ideas and feelings in ways that are appropriate to their age.

Dr. O'Higgins is a great believer in using humor to talk about intimacy. If she is dealing with a group of boys who are giggling because she is talking about blow jobs, she will say yes, it is funny—and then goes on to explain what they are in clear and unembarrassed terms, as well as how not everyone wants to receive or perform them. She talks in a way that is both positive and carefully emphasizes the need for consent.

I was talking to Linsey Blair about this, and she noted that it's sometimes true that in the intention of teachers to be anatomically clear and clinical in conveying physical facts to younger children in sex education classes, they can misjudge the tone. She described a lesson used to help 11- and 12-year-olds understand the biology of sex, where the words used to describe how intercourse happens were "penetration," "ejaculation," "vagina," and "penis," all entirely appropriate, but perhaps scary for some of the children involved. Her view is that sex education should be tackled in smaller groups, where the educators use the natural curiosity of the children to find out what they know or what they think they already know. This would tend to make the session less of a lesson and more of a chat. This doesn't mean adults should shy away from tough questions, but it helps to listen for what the kids are really asking and to respond in a way that matches where they are. Like Dr. O'Higgins, she is a huge believer in humor. "You're trying to have curiosity and encourage their curiosity and get some stuff back," she says. "Sex isn't a concrete block that you're handing to someone and saying, 'This is sex.' I think that still happens sometimes."

My own feeling is that it's incredibly important to be age appropriate in how we talk about sex and intimacy to our children and teenagers, but that encouraging body awareness in a suitable way from a young age might help children and teenagers to understand their own bodies and so their own sexual feelings better. You obviously aren't going to talk about the clitoris or an erect penis to primary school children, but you might want them to be supported in listening to themselves and to be taught the appropriate language to ask for what they want from their teachers, or from their fellow classmates, and to have a sense of their bodies and how they will grow.

I've run a session in junior schools with kids aged 6 to 7 years, where we explore the organs of the body by creating a squishy shape out of cushions and toys, a technique also first encountered at the 2008 Body-Mind Centering workshop run by Mark Chandlee Taylor. I'll bring in a pillowcase and put toys inside that represent the different organs—a bean bag for the liver to show its density and fluffy rabbits for the lungs because they are soft and squishy, and a long snake for the intestines. Once the pillow of body toys has been investigated, we look at building a body of organs out of balloons. I fill some balloons with water or air, at different levels of softness, to represent all of the different organs of the body: heart, lungs, liver, spleen, pancreas, kidneys, bladder, womb, gonads, etc.

After using plastic wrap to hold each part of the body's organs together, for example, the lungs and the heart, and then the liver, kidneys, pancreas, and spleen, etc., you plastic wrap the whole body into shape, until you've got this very compact organ body. Of course, if you lie on one of the balloons it will burst, but when they are all held together inside the plastic wrap, you can lie on them and it gives the youngsters a really lovely, visceral experience of the anatomy of their body, and how everything is connected and how each organ is in support of every other organ. I then get the kids to dance, expressing which organ they like the most.

The company I Heart Guts makes "organ plushies," which are another great resource for engaging young people with their internal organs in an enjoyable way.

As I've said, I took this exercise from Bonnie Bainbridge Cohen's BMC. With older children I might then explore her explanations of what is fundamental to each organ. In her book *Sensing, Feeling, and Action,* she shares people's experiences of their different organs. "They are not absolute edicts but shared personal perceptions," she says. She goes through all the organs—heart, liver, lungs, and so on. She talks about the uterus and vagina as representing the "female organs; vessel of life; feminine, embracing and rejecting; power of giving birth to what one has created; communication; responsiveness; assertiveness; playfulness; accommodating." The prostate and penis on the other hand she describes as "male organ; male extremity; masculinity; communication; responsiveness; power of projecting one's creativity into the world; entering; assertiveness; playfulness; accommodating."[11]

What's interesting to me in terms of how we think about intimacy is that so often the masculine and feminine are presented as oppositional. Bainbridge Cohen on the other hand sees the sexual organs as sharing certain qualities, being accommodating, being playful, and being creative. For both masculine and feminine, you have an idea, a spark of creativity that grows and develops until you give birth to that idea and then make it happen, the spark of creativity going out into the world, to connect and communicate with others, interacting out in the world. I find that rather beautiful.

If you acknowledge that aspects of intimacy are essentially funny, that there is humor to be found in bodies and all their different parts, that begins to take the sense of shame and embarrassment out of the conversation. There are lots of brilliant books, some of which I've listed at the end of the chapter, that help us to talk about sex in a straightforward yet amusing way, acknowledging that it is a good thing to be curious, to see, and to understand. Take, for example, the book *Sex Is a Funny Word,* which seems to me to be a great resource for parents and children aged from 8 to 10 to use as a basis for conversations about sex. It's set out in a comic book format, in bright colors, and allows a young person to engage in the subject matter in a clear, accessible way. It's deliberately inclusive, with children and families of all identities and types. Or there's *Let's Talk About Sex,* now in its twentieth edition, part of the Let's Talk series, which offers accurate and up-to-date guidance for teens and preteens and contains information on puberty, birth control, internet and texting safety, and LGBTQ+ issues, all in a language and pictures that are accessible and engaging.

There are also numerous guides for parents and adults to help them overcome any difficulty they may feel in tackling subjects that can seem sensitive and embarrassing. As my kids were growing up, we had a policy to be truthful whenever they asked anything. If your children ask you something, I think it's important to let them know you are a nonjudgmental resource; answer them with age-appropriate honesty and, if you don't know something, then tell them you will get back to them on the subject and go away and do your own research. In this way, you can help your kids be confident in their own inquisitiveness.

In my own world, even talking to adults, I have found that clarity overcomes embarrassment. I was asked to speak at a film conference recently to share the Intimacy on Set Guidelines, talking both about the creation of onscreen intimacy in straightforward ways, and about the pragmatic professional process in gaining the actor's agreement and consent to the intimate content that they will be asked to perform. Afterward, I was really surprised at how many people came up to me and thanked me for being so direct. I had offered a structure that enabled people to talk expansively and without embarrassment about the creation of intimate encounters.

In talking about intimate scenes in a professional capacity, we are aware not to use language that is objectifying, titillating, or infantilizing. Phrases such as "Come here, babe" or "Hi, darling" are not encouraged. Similarly, when talking about body parts and intimate content, we use language that is adult and professional. For example, saying breasts instead of tits, buttocks not butt, intercourse instead of "give her (or him) a good roll in the hay," penis instead of "your one-eyed trouser snake."

When you are in a relationship, you and your partner can call your body parts whatever you choose, but this is a professional situation in a workplace. In life, in general, it helps to have this clear structure to talk about things in an open and considerate way. It gives people a language beyond the colloquial way to talk about the body. The idea of a positive sexual awakening and being equipped to explore the way our bodies work, and the context of feelings, would, in an ideal world, give teenagers and young people the tools to understand their own growing up, and to have the language and comprehension to be able to call their boundaries. The reason that a series such as *Normal People* had such resonance with young people is that it showed a couple exploring the parameters of their relationship with respect for each other. That's why *Sex Education* struck a chord too.

For example, episode 4 of season 1 dealt with a relationship between two childhood friends who gradually realized that they were both lesbians. As they discovered their sexuality, they entered into a sexual relationship with each other; it failed because one of them wasn't attracted to the other as her sexual partner. The episode showed them finding a way to talk about this; by communicating clearly and openly, they found happiness.

One of the themes of *I May Destroy You* also included the need to be clear and honest. When a gay male character had a one-night stand with a woman without telling her he also had sex with men, his friends confronted him about his lack of honesty, warning him that he should have been open so that the woman could make an informed choice. Both are examples of teaching young people about the need to speak openly about sex and consent.

Filmed encounters such as these suggest that if youngsters are conscious of physical, emotional, and psychological factors in their behavior, they can make responsible, reasonable, positive choices. One person might opt for a casual sexual encounter, another might commit to a long-term relationship. These choices and everything in between are all fine provided they are explored with mutual respect, agreement, and consent.

I recognize that there are a lot of balancing acts here. When sexual educators such as Dr. O'Higgins go into schools, they always work with parents because they recognize their important role in their children's upbringing. The sex education schools provide needs the backing and the reinforcement of parents if it is to succeed. This supports the parents in having an insight into what and how the Active* Consent program will be delivered, encouraging open communication from the parent to the pupil and the school. Parents feel relieved saying things like "It's given me more confidence to approach this topic with my son!" or "I love the way you show sex in such a positive way to young people, when it occurs in a loving consensual manner," and "I now know that I owe it to my son (for his safety and happiness) to have this conversation with him."

Nevertheless, in my experience, while it is healthy for parents to be open with their children, it is also true that at some point, teenagers don't want their parents to be the person they confide in. They may need another trusted adult around who they can talk to—perhaps a teacher, or perhaps another relative or friend. They don't want to, and they don't have to, share everything with their parents as they grow to adulthood. It is right and proper for teenagers to separate themselves from their parents as they move into adulthood in order to establish a rite of passage. That is why talking about sex in a positive and age-appropriate way with an independent adult who you trust can be so important.

My feeling is that in much of the world, our education is

still quite Victorian in outlook. It's a model that dictates to children rather than listening to them and working out what information to share.

I believe very passionately in an education system that aims to nurture our children and teenagers. I hope it might help them to become young people who have the emotional and verbal skills to make informed decisions about how they are in themselves and in their relationships, and then give them the language in which they can ask for that in a respectful way.

If I'm really talking about utopia, I'd like us as a society to be asking ourselves what we can put in place in our primary and junior schools to support children in knowing that their instincts are valid and respected and to give them appropriate language to ask for what they want, be it from a teacher, one of their friends, or a parent. Girls are starting to experience puberty and begin menstruating much younger than in the past. Boys are masturbating at primary school level, and many will already have encountered some pornographic or explicit sexual images. Ideally, we need to support children to understand the basics of their bodies and how they work before they leave junior school. But we also need to go beyond biology and encourage them to understand that what they feel about themselves is valuable, so they are equipped with a strong sense of self as they enter secondary school, and can call their boundaries and say what upsets or confuses them. For those nurturing our young people, be it as a parent or teacher, we need to educate ourselves in how to speak to them and be active listeners so that they will see us as a nonjudgmental resource.

I'm a great believer, as I've made clear in the earlier

chapters, in improving connection to the natural world to support a healthy life. The same need for groundedness and mindfulness is true for our children, teenagers, and young people when learning about the world and in education. Life can be enhanced by the outdoors. In many countries, such as Sweden, outdoor learning is common practice. In the UK, a number of forest schools based on the policy of Swedish outdoor education have been established. The more we anchor our children and teenagers in their bodies and nurture their connection with nature, the more they can feel their place in the world and in their relationships. This could be supported by activities such as yoga and mindfulness taught in age-appropriate ways for kids in infant and junior schools.

In a different context, it is very often the case that when children are touched inappropriately or abused in some way, they know what is happening to them is wrong. Trained counselors and psychologists have learned that it is important to take children at their word and investigate what is happening to them.

I tend to believe that children have good instincts. As parents, it's all too easy to say, "Oh, go on, give your granny a kiss," or, "Why don't you hug Uncle Arthur?" and to force children to do that when they are reluctant. But they might have good reasons for their hesitation. Granny might not smell very nice, or she might be unkind when you are not looking. Uncle Arthur perhaps has anger issues. Or maybe, there is some form of inappropriate behavior going on that we don't know about. My belief is that we should listen to our children and respect that they are calling their boundaries when they don't want to hug someone.

It's a way of teaching them fundamental respect for

themselves, allowing them to respond to feelings that they may not always be able to express. For me, this basic respect is a way of eliciting positive behavior in children, teenagers, and young people, by supporting them to take ownership of how they feel and revealing that they can draw a line in how they are going to respond.

There will always be cultural differences in how these conversations take place. It's one thing for an agnostic parent to respond to a child's question about where babies come from, and another for someone from a strictly religious culture with different traditions. But I wonder whether attempting to ground sexual education in respect and openness might offer a way forward. If you are encouraging each young person within their family, within their restraints, to listen to themselves, then they can choose what to take on board. They might choose to observe cultural or religious traditions, or they might break with those. But you're helping them to make the choice that is right for them.

If a young person is within a constrained culture or religion, positive sex education seems a better way to give them information than the porn sites and social media that they turn to because they are too embarrassed to talk to their parents, teachers, or peers.

One of the other things I found fascinating in my discussions with Dr. O'Higgins is her work in explaining the difference between the physiology of arousal and actual desire. The workshops for Active* Consent look at three real-life scenarios and ask teenagers what they could have said or done during a sexual encounter to gain consent that is OMFG (ongoing, mutual, and freely given) to achieve a better outcome to the narrative. In one, a boy forces a girl to give him a blow job after she has smiled at him at a party. In another, a couple have oral sex and then meet a few days later, and one says they do not want to be intimate again. Both are about helping young people find better ways to communicate.

The third scenario involves a couple where the woman forces the man to have sex. It attempts to increase understanding of physiology, to explain how a woman's body will lubricate to protect itself from damage, even when she is being raped, and that a man may get an erection even though he doesn't want to have sex. It describes the difference between the physiology of arousal and desire. This physical phenomenon is called arousal nonconcordance, and occurs when your body's physiological response to something doesn't match your psychological feelings of desire. Chapter Six of Emily Nagoski's book *Come As You Are* charts this clearly and gives excellent insight into understanding something that can be both confusing and upsetting.

This is important when it comes to understanding the effects of pornography. A 9-year-old boy may be aroused by watching pornography, but it doesn't mean he desires to have sex. A 20-year-old may get an erection watching strangulation, but that doesn't indicate that that is the way that desires to he have intercourse with his girlfriend.

Pornography and the sexual images so widely circulated on social media objectify bodies. Exposure to those images is making our young people see each other as sexual objects rather than human beings. It separates them, and sometimes separates them far too young, from the idea that the person is someone they know, someone who has their own needs and desires. It conditions them to see each other as bodies rather than whole individuals. This is antithetical to the idea of intimacy, which is about connection between people in all their unique complexities.

In 2023's *Barbie,* directed by Greta Gerwig, Ken discovers that in the real world, women are objects to be belittled—just as Kens are in the Barbie world. Underneath the fun and laughter, Gerwig is offering a serious critique of misogyny and objectification. The moral of the film is that everyone should be respected for who they are as a whole being, not for how they look or the role they play. It is an important lesson delivered in a pink-wrapped package, and it is what I advocate for to be part of every young person's education.

When I am training intimacy practitioners, I always ask them about how they hold the space, how they create a safe space, how they hold themselves in the room in order to encourage and support people to share. They often talk about listening well, asking questions, leaning forward into the space. But in many ways, it is about the opposite. You need to pull back so you create a space within which someone can experience themselves.

It's not about telling people and imposing but about turning yourself into the universal listener, allowing the other person to discover what they need to say. I was really touched that when I worked with Andrew Garfield on *We Live in Time,* he gave an interview in which he showed how deeply he had understood that creation of space. He said: "There was something immediately boundary-making about it—we were suddenly given a really firm playpen by [Ita] who was creative, sensitive and clear. We knew that if there were any issue, that issue was going to be very, very short lived . . . You need to make sure that everyone feels safe."[12]

Making sure that everyone feels safe is part of the ideal sex education in our schools, giving our children and teenagers a really clear playpen within which they can explore their sexual awakening and expression. If sexual education is built on open communication, understanding, agreement and consent, and mutual pleasure to support them in their sexual awakening, not on fear and silence, it will begin to help to counter the ocean of misunderstanding that our teenagers and young people are awash in today. The lessons I have learned in my practice, along with the insights brilliant sex educators are bringing into our classrooms, feel like a better way forward.

AGE-APPROPRIATE BOOKS . . .

RESOURCES FOR PARENTS AND FOR CHILDREN AND YOUNG PEOPLE ON BODIES AND RELATIONSHIPS

As parents, it's our job to teach our children about sex. We all hope that our children will grow into good people "at home in their own skins" with warm hearts and having the knowledge and strength to survive and thrive. Beyond "the talk," which covers biology and reproduction, there is more we can say about the human experience of being in our bodies.

There are a lot of resources out there and what follows is a short list of books, websites, and even a couple of interesting TED Talks with ideas that are for the most part reliable and unbiased sources of information that you as a parent can use to add to your own font of knowledge and choose which parts and when to share those insights with your children.

Parenthood can be an exciting journey, not one worry after another, as it's so often portrayed.

Ideas for Parents

Books

- *Raising Boys in the 21st Century and Raising Girls in the 21st Century* by Steve Biddulph

- Biddulph's two books are both guides and a call-to-arms for parents; they are powerful, practical, and positive. The five key stages of girlhood and three of boyhood are laid out so that you know exactly what matters at which age, and how to build strength and connectedness into your children from infancy onward. All the hazards are signposted—bullying, eating disorders, body image, depression, social media harms and helps—as are concrete and simple measures for parents to help prevent their children from becoming victims.

- *Boys & Sex* and *Girls & Sex* by Peggy Orenstein

- Drawing on in-depth interviews with young people and a wide range of psychologists, academics, and experts, Peggy Orenstein explores often hidden truths, hard lessons, and important possibilities of our young people's sex lives in the modern world. She gives comprehensive and in-depth information with which to understand, and navigate, this complicated new world.

- *BoyMom: Reimagining Boyhood in the Age of Impossible Masculinity* by Ruth Whippman

- *BoyMom* is about what it means to grow up male in an era when #MeToo has zeroed our tolerance for toxic masculinity, yet the pressure on young men to be "masculine" has never been more intense. It is also a mother's story. As a feminist mom of three sons, Ruth Whippman is all too aware that her parenting today will shape the men her sons become tomorrow, but daily life can often feel like the triumph of nature over nurture. Empathetic, witty, and curious, *BoyMom* asks how we can give boys a healthier, more expansive story about their own lives.

- *Sex Education Answer Book* by Cath Hakanson
- Includes child-friendly answers to more than 200 commonly asked questions. The content is organized by age group and helps parents build confidence to speak to their children about reproduction, sex, bodies, relationships, pregnancy, masturbation, sexual diversity, gender, STIs, and more.

- *Going Beyond "The Talk": Relationships and Sexuality Education for Those Supporting 12–18 Year Olds* by Sanderijn van der Doof, Clare Bennett, and Arris Lueks

- The book explores the challenges in adult-child communication about sexuality and provides helpful advice on how to establish an open and positive dialogue, covering topics like social media, porn, and sexual development in UK, US, and Australian contexts. Specific age-based guidance for 12-year-olds to older teens. Throughout, the book emphasizes the importance of positive sexuality education, empowering young people to make their own choices on how to enjoy their relationships and sexuality in a safe and consensual way.

Two Interesting TED Talks

- Sue Jaye Johnson: What We Don't Teach Kids About Sex | TED Talk

- Emily Quinn: The Way We Think About Biological Sex Is Wrong | TED Talk

Two Interesting and Useful Websites

- Sexualwellbeing.ie—helping to turn the big talk into many little talks
- Scarleteen.com—for teenagers

Books for Children and Teenagers

For younger children:

- *Mummy Laid an Egg!* by Babette Cole
- In this story the children put their embarrassed parents straight and dispel the myths surrounding baby-making, growth, and birth. A no-nonsense text with funny illustrations.
- *What Makes a Baby* by Cory Silverberg and Fiona Smyth
- It is a twenty-first-century children's picture book about conception, gestation, and birth, which reflects the reality of our modern time by being inclusive of all kinds of kids, adults, and families, regardless of how many people are involved, their orientation, gender and other identity, or family composition. Just as important, the story doesn't gender people or body parts, so most parents and families will find that it leaves room for them to educate their child without having to erase their own experience.

- *Love Makes a Family (It's Cool to Be Kind)* by Sophie Beer

- Whether a child has two moms, two dads, one parent, or one of each, this simple preschool read-aloud demonstrates that what's most important in each family's life is the love the family members share.

- *Hair in Funny Places* by Babette Cole

- This picture book uses a similar approach to *Mummy Laid an Egg* to explain puberty.

- *Let's Talk About Sex* by Robie H. Harris

- This book is a classic sexual health resource designed primarily for preteens and teens, but it also serves as an excellent guide for parents, teachers, and anyone who cares about a young person's sexual well-being. The book provides accurate, updated information on a range of topics, from puberty and conception to birth control and the internet's impact, all presented in an approachable way to answer questions and help young people make responsible decisions

- *Wait, What?: A Comic Book Guide to Relationships, Bodies, and Growing Up* by Heather Corinna and Isabella Rotman

- A graphic narrative guide that covers essential topics for preteens and young teens about their changing bodies and feelings. Using comics, activities, and examples, a group of friends give encouragement and context for new and confusing feelings and experiences.

- *Welcome to Your Period!* by Yumi Stynes and Dr. Melissa Kang
- Offers honest advice and big-sisterly wisdom on all the things girls need to know: from what cramps feel like to whether you can feel blood coming out, to what you should do if your pad leaks onto your clothes.
- *Sex Is a Funny Word* by Corey Silverberg
- *Sex Is a Funny Word* is a comic book that teaches sex education to those aged 8–10. What makes the book so special is its inclusivity; it features children and families of every race, gender-identity, and sexual orientation. Much more than a simple "facts of life" or "the birds and the bees" book, it opens up conversations between young people and their caregivers in a way that allows adults to convey their values and beliefs while providing information about boundaries, safety, and joy.
- *The Gender Book* by Mel Reift Hill and Jay Mays
- A colorful, all-ages visual primer on the world of gender. Based on research with more than 300 questionnaires and dozens of one-on-one interviews with members of the communities depicted, this book represents an agreement of many diverse community voices and a huge step forward in the world of gender education.
- *S.E.X., Second Edition: The All-You-Need-to-Know Sexuality Guide to Get You Through Your Teens and Twenties* by Heather Corinna

- As a teenager or emerging adult, dealing with all the changes going on in your life, body, and mind can be mighty overwhelming. When it comes to sex, everyone seems to have strong feelings and opinions about who you should be and what you should (shouldn't) do. *S.E.X.* clearly spells out what you need and want to know—no shame, no judgment, just comprehensive and accurate information in clear, straightforward language.

- *Sex and Lovers: A Practical Guide* by Ann-Marlene Henning and Tina Bremer-Olszewski

- This book exposes the deceits of pornography and talks about common fears and pressures to perform. With a really accessible text for teenagers upward, *Sex and Lovers* asks and answers masses of questions in an honest, straightforward, and entirely open manner. Specially commissioned photographs are truthful and authentic and the opposite of the voyeuristic images purveyed by pornography.

CHAPTER TEN

A LIFETIME OF INTIMATE RELATIONSHIPS

As we make our way as adults in the world, how do we navigate our desires as our search for intimacy and love opens out to the challenges of adult life? How do we balance the concepts of listening to ourselves, doing what is right for us, exploring our fantasies, finding love, calling our boundaries, and listen to our partner's needs, desires, and their boundaries? How do we give love and accept being loved in a healthy way? And, in longer-term relationships, how do we evolve and grow with our partners as time changes us, as we move through the shifting hormonal cycles of life?

I always feel a certain irony when I stand up in front of people to talk about intimacy and simulated sex scenes, or when I sit quietly in a room with two actors and a director and offer choreographic suggestions as to how they might simulate orgasm. As I've explained in earlier chapters, this openness about sex is the antithesis of the way I was brought up. I come from a strictly traditional Irish Catholic family, where talking about sex and intimacy was just not on the agenda. My mother was a midwife, but that didn't mean she was at all open about bodily functions. I can still remember how embarrassed she was when I asked her to help me to use a tampon when I had my first period.

I'm not a therapist or a sexual educator. But life has a habit of making us experts in fields that we don't expect. Take Dakota Johnson. She starred in one of the most famous twenty-first-century depictions of intimacy onscreen.[1] When E. L. James's erotic bestseller *Fifty Shades of Grey*, about the sado-masochistic relationship between an innocent student and handsome billionaire, was made into a film in 2015 directed by Sam Taylor-Johnson (no relation to Dakota), Dakota was cast as the naïve Anastasia opposite Jamie Dornan as Christian Grey.

I met Dakota when I was taking part in the panel discussion on intimacy at Sundance Film Festival in 2023 and was impressed by her commitment to the cause of making sexual well-being central to how we view life through her involvement with the company maude. This modern sexual wellness company, founded by Éva Goicochea, is "on a mission to make intimacy better— for all people . . . When we set out to create a modern intimacy brand, we saw an industry long overdue for change. We wanted to create sexual wellness products that could be truly integrated into your world."[2] With the company's idea of making sexual agency better and providing gender-neutral sexual well-being tools and toys that are deliberately designed to be different from the gaudy vibrators and sexual aids more widely available, maude reflects the cultural shifts that have gone on ever since the #MeToo revelations that emerged just as the company was founded.

Intimacy coordinators on set were part of that journey. "I've actually never worked with an intimacy coordinator," Dakota said. "That didn't exist when I did my big naked franchise [*Fifty Shades of Grey*]. I was just kind of thrown to the wolves on that one." She went on to praise the level of care that is now brought to such vulnerable moments as "extremely smart and definitely kind of parallel with what the global conversation [around sex] is." Then she paused. "Well, maybe not global. But we'll get there."[3]

It was interesting to me that the actor so specifically linked her own unprotected journey through the graphic depiction of intimacy onscreen with her desire to alter the landscape of intimacy in our lives. *Fifty Shades of Grey* seemed as if it was groundbreaking in its intimate content in its day, but it was concerning in the nature of intimacy and the questionable aspect of consent in its depiction of BDSM sexual play.

What's lovely about what Dakota and Éva are doing with the ethos of maude is that it allows us to embrace pleasure. By normalizing our access to aids for physical intimacy, the company allows people to bring new qualities to their sexual play. They don't have to go to sex shops, or to stumble upon pornography when they try to buy vaginal moisturizers or vibrators online. Everything is upfront and clear. This enables people to stay present, curious, and open. It frees sex and sexual exploration from any sense of embarrassment; it is helping to bring about attitudes that are far healthier.

I feel that my own journey has also been part of that process. If we are going to improve our intimate relations, then perhaps we need to find a way of thinking and understanding that starts in consent, communication, and honesty. As I've researched more, I've come to understand that sustaining intimacy through our lives requires a level of openness and transparency that can be challenging to achieve. Understanding intimacy, shedding shame, and building stronger connections within ourselves and with our partners is an ongoing process. How many of us consciously know what motivates and drives us, where our blocks and fears lie, how deep in our psyche we play out familial patterns? The reason people approach therapists and counselors, such as Linsey Blair or Dr. Orla Guralnik, about their intimate relations is because therapists can offer a deep dive into an understanding of why we do what we do, and what unconscious patterns are driving our behavior. Very often sexual issues arise from people's hopes, fears, or expectations not being met, and those feelings often grow from things that have happened when someone is growing up, and an individual's own relationship with their parents and with their parenting.

I was talking to Linsey Blair, for example, about the way that onscreen, and in novels and plays for that matter, there's a constant idea of instant attraction. Eyes meet across a crowded room and, wham, people are immediately in love. Biologically this probably has some truth in it, especially when you are young. The male of the species is on the lookout for a suitable mate who will continue their line, and they respond to obvious signals in terms of body and attraction as I've discussed. In a similar way, the female is looking for a male with strong genes who can protect and provide.

Psychologically, however, if you're looking for a long-term intimate relationship, that spontaneous mutual attraction, which feels so good, may actually be an unconscious attraction to something familiar—and that might not be a good thing. As Blair explains: "If you've come from a poor attachment background, which might even contain neglect or abuse, then you might go 'ping' with someone from a very similar background, which may lead to repeated failures in relationships."

She told me about a woman she had counseled who had a father with undiagnosed mental health issues; every man she felt an immediate kinship with also, eventually, turned out to have similar undiagnosed mental health issues. Yet that was the excitement she sought. When she went on dates with men who were relatively well-adjusted, she found them boring. In that instance, Blair suggested she ignore the initial spark and try to deliberately build a bond with someone whom she hadn't experienced that instant rapport and attraction with. With time and effort, she met someone with whom she could develop a healthier relationship. That big fantasy of finding "the one" was replaced, in real life, by a willingness to work on attraction and to build desire.

The positive takeaway is that she put time and effort into understanding her unconscious patterns and worked with a therapist to support her to create more healthy relationships. And when she did develop a healthier relationship, she was willing to put the work into nurturing and growing that relationship.

As I mentioned in Chapter Three, I once read an article in the *New York Times* about the influential study in which the psychologist Dr. Arthur Aron claimed to lead two people to fall in love in a laboratory.[4] He invited a heterosexual man and woman to sit face to face and answer 36 increasingly personal questions. Then they stared silently into one another's eyes for four minutes. People latched on to the experiment because it seemed to work; the subjects who answered the 36 questions ended up much closer than the couples who engaged in small talk for the same period. What's more, six months later, the two participants were married and invited the entire laboratory to the ceremony.

It would be naïve to think that asking and answering questions creates love or causes people to fall in love (as Linsey Blair points out, there are always unconscious factors in play that are unmeasurable and unknowable in both parties). But the actual act of sharing personal information with someone who shares back can create a feeling of intimacy.

Three things really interest me about the study. The first is that the questions are based on finding a degree of commonality between two people; they are looking to find attitudes that they share, and Dr. Aron's questions speed up that process, propelling people into a vulnerability and an openness that might normally take weeks or months to build. The second is that the study formalizes the idea of the gaze changing and deepening your opinion of someone.

A version of the 36 questions can be used as an acting tool. One of my colleagues, Miranda Harcourt, a renowned acting coach who regularly works with Nicole Kidman, among many others, has written about the way in which these questions can be used as "an approach that can achieve true connection in a short space of time." She actually talked to Dr. Aron about using his system in this way when she was working on the film *Lost Girls* in 2020.

"Dr. Aron's claim is that mutual vulnerability fosters closeness. One key pattern associated with the development of a close relationship among peers is sustained, reciprocal, personal self-disclosure." Harcourt "used elements of this exercise as a basis to create relationships between lovers, between parents, between best friends, or between siblings" in her acting coaching work.[5]

I haven't used them myself, but an intimacy practitioner whom I had mentored used them on a production where actors were playing a married couple. First, they went through the questions as themselves, omitting any they didn't want to answer since they were not trying to spark a real-life relationship. (Some of the questions are too invasive to use as a professional tool.) In this way, they quickly got to know one another on a personal basis, short-circuiting social chitchat. Later, when they were up to speed with their characters, they repeated the questions in character, which enabled them to make discoveries about the fictional relationship.

The third thing that fascinates me about Dr. Aron's study is that the process is an active one. The author of the *New York Times* piece, Canadian author Mandy Len Catron, ended up saying exactly that. "What I like about this study is how it assumes that love is an action. It assumes that what matters to my partner matters to me because we have at least three things in common . . . It's true you can't choose who loves you . . . and you can't create romantic feelings based on convenience alone. Science tells us biology matters; our pheromones and hormones do a lot of work behind the scenes. But despite all this, I've begun to think love is a more pliable thing than we make it out to be.

Arthur Aron's study taught me that it's possible—simple, even—to generate trust and intimacy, the feelings love needs to thrive."

The acknowledgment that open sharing is the basis for an ongoing relationship is worth always remembering. Intimate relationships hit little turning points all the time. Moving beyond the hook-up is a crucial next stage in every relationship. Then, if things develop, there might be another point of change when a couple has children. Later, after the children leave home, and women go through menopause, there are more alterations required. Intimacy alters over the course of our lives, yet quite often we stay on the same script, using the things that worked in the past to give us pleasure in the present.

I'd definitely like us to be much more open in the way that we approach the radical changes that women's bodies go through—not just over years, but every month. I've talked in an earlier chapter about how groundbreaking I felt the treatment of menstruation was in *I May Destroy You*, where it wasn't something to be ashamed of but simply a part of life. I worked more recently on a historical drama where the producers and writers worked with the historian Ruth Goodman because they wanted to include an accurate depiction of how figures in the past coped with their monthly bleed, using rolled up strips of old linen and other old cloth rags—hence the phrase "on the rag."

This historical accuracy goes beyond simple information. It helps to create a context where the monthly cycle of ovulation isn't seen as a problem, but as something that is intrinsic to the cycle of women's desire. It helps foster an understanding that hormones rise as you are about to ovulate, and that women's intimate lives are often affected by the emotional flows generated by their bodily functions. If those cycles are acknowledged, they are powerful, not shaming. One of the persistent challenges I have found in my work is that—perhaps because the medical profession is so predominantly male—there is still a huge amount of shame and secrecy, lack of information, and confusion surrounding perfectly normal and natural bodily functions, such as periods and menopause.

Red School is an organization that describes itself as "rooted in the bloody, wild, radical power of the menstrual cycle."[6] In their 2017 book, *Wild Power: Discover the Magic of Your Menstrual Cycle and Awaken the Feminine Path to Power,* the authors and founders Alexandra Pope and Sjanie Hugo Wurlitzer shift a woman's relationship with her menstrual cycle by likening it to the seasons, where each part of the cycle is different but necessary. They suggest that by understanding the gift that each part of the cycle gives, you can work with its power. It's not a curse, or something to be vilified, but an energy to be embraced, celebrated, and explored.

Periods signify women's role as child-bearers, and another thing we don't see much of onscreen is empowering depictions of birth. They are there but often treated as a moment of comedy or, in contrast, extreme and frightening pain. Yet birth is a natural process, something women were designed to do, and the most incredible experience for many of them. In *We Live in Time,* a love story, directed by John Crowley, that's both life-affirming and deeply moving, Florence Pugh and Andrew Garfield play a loving couple, Almut and Tobias, whose relationship has been shaped by illness and childlessness.

When Almut finally gets pregnant, through IVF, she ends

up giving birth in a disabled toilet in a petrol service station. It was a wonderful scene to work on, choreographed with the help of a specialist midwife, Penny Taylor, to support John, Florence, and Andrew. We were all focused on bringing fundamental truth to the portrayal of this scene. Tobias is talked through the stages and the support needed to deliver the baby by a midwife on the telephone, while Almut is on her hands and knees, present in the intensity of labor.

The scene is the precise opposite from the kind of 2-D depictions of women that I've talked about in previous chapters, where we are used to seeing women's fragmented bodies, not embodied in space, infantilized by lighting that washes them out and hides their wrinkles. This is a moment when we see a woman's body in all its incredibleness, full-frame, in relationship with her partner at the moment of giving birth. It's a celebration of all that power and glory, and of a new life.

That new life is amazing, but it is also a transformative moment that once again changes the script of intimacy. Take the moment after a couple have had children. There's a really good book called *Life After Birth: What Even Your Friends Won't Tell You About Motherhood* by Kate Figes and Jean Zimmerman that makes it clear just how difficult it is to renegotiate the dynamic with your partner when you are new parents, let alone continue to find intimate moments for the two of you after children have arrived in your life.[7] One important aspect of that is to acknowledge and discuss the way in which, during the process of birth, a woman's body and her genitalia go from being a very private place, known only to her and her partner, to a functional part of the anatomy, open to everyone who happens to be involved in the act of giving birth.

When I supported the scene in *We Live in Time*, I was very aware to make sure that the characters working as the gas-station attendants averted their eyes to give Pugh's character some privacy. But anyone who has given birth knows how strange a state it is, often with multiple professionals around you, midwives, doctors, and so on. For many couples, the aftermath of this sudden change in how you both view the birth giver can be one of the biggest transformations you face when you become a parent. If the woman chooses to breastfeed, her breasts that might formerly have been a source of sensual pleasure suddenly become functional. Tiredness is another factor to navigate and negotiate in keeping your sex life active as you adjust to this period of your relationship. According to the National Childbirth Trust, "It can take time to feel like having sex again after birth. A positive approach could involve patience, a sense of humor, understanding, and a willingness to find new ways of expressing physical affection until you both feel ready to have sex again."[8]

The same might be true after one person in a relationship has had an operation and their body is suddenly unfamiliar and different, not responding to caresses or erotic stimuli in quite the same way. Equally, illnesses such as cancer or dementia can have a profound effect on intimate relationships, bringing their own challenges and concerns, for both parties. For example, Rose Ryan works with people with Parkinson's and has commented, "We know that anxiety and stress cuts through desire like a knife . . . What turns us on is if we see ourselves reflected as beautiful in our partners eyes." She goes on to say, "Intimacy and sex are dynamic through the journey of our relationships; things that worked once and felt good might need to be changed . . . Negotiation and adaptability are vital . . . "[9] As Linsey Blair points out, long-term relationships can suffer from a death of curiosity. We assume we know the other person completely. In the same way established couples finish each other's sentences, so in intimate terms they assume they know what the other person is thinking, and it can all get a bit boring. A conversation, a chat, about what each of you are feeling never goes amiss.

When she is talking to couples who are worrying about their intimate lives, Blair suggests they write a fantasy together, like a chapter of a book that they expect someone else to read. It has to be written from the heart, with characters moving from first meeting to sexual intercourse, to postcoital intimacy. Writing in this way can make people feel shy and exposed. But so much emerges about what they actually want in a relationship. It helps them to talk and to discuss their desires in a frame. One might want to get the blindfold out; another might simply want to talk. By exploring their separate fantasies, they perhaps create space to laugh and joke, to find a way to mutual satisfaction.

Another way to communicate is to concentrate not on sexual intercourse, but on sensuous touch and contact. Most couples could benefit from setting aside time simply to be together and touch one another. With increasing numbers of us working from home, the danger is that in longer-term relationships, we mistake familiarity for intimacy. Because we are working and living alongside each other, we assume we are making a connection, yet we are not really engaging with each other, let alone creating intimacy.

It's worth remembering at this point that not all closeness in personal relationships is physical. It is possible to have intimacy without sex and sex without intimacy. Emotional, intellectual, experiential, and even spiritual bonds are just as important as physical ones and can be cultivated in similar ways. They require trust and vulnerability from two people, an approach to one another that is based in compassion and genuine care. They require us to listen as well as to speak, to share our innermost feelings but also to listen carefully and respectfully.

Actually, being present in a shared space is key to all forms of intimacy. When we first meet someone, we may spend hours in a pub gazing into each other's eyes, whispering sweet nothings, just relishing being in one another's company. That kind of intense romantic gaze is probably deeply irritating to the people around us, but it is profoundly good for our intimate lives, both physical and emotional.

In fact, spending time connecting with your partner gazing into their eyes is a beautiful gift to each other at every point in our relationships, and every age of our lives. When you see a 2-year-old walking down the street, they stop at every flower and every crack in the sidewalk and really notice the world. As an adult, you walk down the same street and the same flowers are there, the same cracks in the pavement, but you just take them for granted. It's the same with looking at a fellow human being. Just pausing and sitting and being present and mindful allows you time and space to see and be with another person, allowing you to drop and connect with your relationship in that moment, be it a parent, friend, or lover.

That close attention to one another is a way of getting around so many of the problems of the contemporary world that put up barriers between us. Our increasing reliance on screens means that society as a whole is missing the softness of touch, that pat on the shoulder, the goodbye hug that embraces you and makes you feel part of the world. I'd suggest that this is an area of our relationships to work on consciously, expanding touch, setting time aside for a mutual massage, or simply sitting next to someone, holding hands, being conscious and mindful with each other.

In the same way, we can experience the joy of waking up our own bodies. Our skin is the largest erogenous organ of the body, and touch makes it come alive in different ways. Engaging in a massage can be the most wonderful sensuous gift. When massaging your partner, you can touch, lick, pound, or caress the skin; you can stimulate erogenous zones such as the nipples. You may have shared what you would like to do previously and then explore the massage in silence or to music. It can also be exciting and sexy to encourage your partner, to explain to them what you feel when they touch different areas of your body or give you oral pleasure. Being explicit about the physical sensations you are experiencing both helps the other person know what you want but is also joyful in itself. The book *The Tao of Sexual Massage* by Stephen Russell and Jürgen Kolb is full of wonderful massages such as "opening the gate of the spine," "mixing the original and joyous fires," "opening the doors of the crimson palace," and "awakening the dragon." It is a really wonderful journey through intimate touch and connection with your partner.

Another positive way to connect with your partner is partner yoga, where the shared postures allow you to connect with the breath and heat of your partner, and to find release together. There is a wonderful book called *Partner Yoga: Making Contact for Physical, Emotional, and Spiritual Growth* by Cain Carroll and Lori Kimata, which "blends mutually beneficial postures, conscious breathing, trust, communication, and—most of all—playfulness and fun . . . *Partner Yoga* is perfect for anyone—novice or seasoned yoga practitioner—who is interested in increasing fitness, releasing tension, strengthening relationships, and having a good time."[10]

It's also true that there are endless books and helpful aids available to improve and deepen your intimate life. There is a lot of great information out there on the internet, but if you worry about coming across pornography while searching for advice, then the development of the sexual wellness industry means there are plenty of places to go to get information. I've listed some helpful and interesting sources starting on page 345.

Like anything else, our intimate relations are something we can constantly engage with and learn about. If we want to play tennis, then perhaps we will watch some YouTube tutorials, read a few manuals, and then—if we are struggling—go for a few private lessons. I'd like to see a world where our attitude to sex and relationships follows that pattern, and where everyone feels they can access helpful, straightforward, non-pornographic information that would help them experience happier intimate relationships throughout their lives. You might not want to go to a tantric sex workshop in order to find more fulfilling physical relations; it would be lovely if there were workshops available for every level of exploration though.

To keep the tennis analogy going, no one assumes that they can just play tennis without any training or guidance. What's more, once they are playing tennis, then they will adapt their game to the opponent they are playing against. The same moves don't work with everyone. It is the same with sex. There is no right or wrong way to have sex, no magical method. Instead, it's helpful to think of our intimate relationships as an evolving game, an experience that will change with time, depending on both our partner's and our own age. If we keep reapplying the same formula no matter the person opposite us, no matter the length of time we've been with them, then it's possible that it will stop working and stop making us happy. We don't keep repeating in the same way in any other walk of life. Why do we do it with our sexual relations?

Attitudes to intimacy have changed over time, most notably since the advent of widely available and safe birth control in the 1960s. As Philip Larkin puts it in the famous opening line to "Annus Mirabilis": *"Sexual intercourse began / In nineteen sixty-three / (which was rather late for me)—/ Between the end of the Chatterley ban / And the Beatles' first LP."* At the same time, as social attitudes evolve and change, the scientific understanding of our bodies and the models on which sexual activity are measured keep altering too.

Individual attitudes to intimacy are likely to be shaped by the ideas current when a person is coming into their sexual awakening. The generations following 1972 may well have on their bookshelves a copy of Alex Comfort's

The Joy of Sex, with its famous line drawings of a woman and a bearded man, talking about sexual techniques in nonmedical but helpful ways.

Its basic message was that couples should experiment and have fun. It offered a menu of possibilities in a cookbook style, with sections including Starters, Main Courses, and Sauces & Pickles. It also emphasized love and care between couples, suggesting that there were no rules as long as people were engaged in sexual activity that they enjoyed and that made them both feel good.

Updated editions have been published ever since the 1970s, and however old-fashioned the drawings may now look, in many ways the work's mantra is still incredibly helpful and liberating. Crucially, I think, it introduces the element of play into our intimate relationships. As I've said in earlier chapters, I think play is an important part of keeping intimate relationships alive. It takes us back to the idea of *le jeu*, that flirtatious creation of a bond between two people. It might just be a question of dancing in the kitchen or stroking one another's backs or tickling each other's feet. But it is an intimate act that can keep a flame alive. The relish of life together and the enjoyment of one another's bodies is easy to lose, yet it feels important to preserve.

I always like the scene I supported for *Normal People* where Connell and Marianne meet after a time apart, when they have both been with other sexual partners. Their coming together is tentative and tender. He kisses her belly as she steps out of the shower, and the gesture initiates the intimacy between them. He is present with her and she with him and from that presence a sexual encounter grows. It seems to me it's important not to endgame intimate relationships in life; you are enjoying each moment for what it is.

In the same way, self-pleasure can be an intimate act. Just as intimacy isn't always about sex, so self-pleasure isn't exactly the same as masturbation. It might lead to masturbation—and it is very healthy for people to have orgasms regularly as it releases "feel good" hormones such as dopamine and endorphins that are really good for you. But it is also about celebrating your body, of finding ways to make yourself feel good.

What's interesting to me is that when you read up about self-pleasure, there is a distinct difference between the advice given to men and women. Type "self-pleasure with a vulva" into the internet, and it is all about candles and soft music, as well as some advice on how to stimulate the clitoris, useful sex toys and lubricants. If you type in "self-pleasure with a penis," the advice given is much more physical and mechanical, generally simply offering masturbation tips.

It's often the same when men present themselves to a doctor with erectile dysfunction. Instead of being offered advice about their intimate life, they are most likely to be prescribed Viagra. It's as if intimacy for men is principally mechanical, an issue that can be solved with technical advice. In an ideal world, why shouldn't men be able to focus on sensual pleasure while women are given really good technical tips? Why shouldn't each inform the other?

An ideal world is what we are talking about here, and I'd like to see our intimate lives much more influenced by an equality that explores different qualities but gives them equal weight. I've always been inspired by the book

Women Who Run with the Wolves: Contacting the Power of the Wild Woman by Clarissa Pinkola Estés, which argues that feminine wildness is a positive and necessary quality for women to carry and cultivate.

Estés says that women's genuine nature has been "repressed for centuries by a value system that trivializes emotional truth, intuitive wisdom and self-confidence." By reveling in our wild nature, we not only reclaim and rejoice in our true feminine power but allow men to exercise the very different qualities of masculine power. It argues for women and men to both be honored and respected for their different attributes, living in a harmony based on what they can both bring to relationships and to life. Women don't have to work in a masculine way in order to be deemed successful and vice versa. Each works within their power and their experience. It's all about balance rather than control.

In the end, keeping sexual activity and intimacy alive through the different stages of life comes back to this balance, underpinned by choice, consent, and conversation. Sometimes people want one thing, sometimes they want another. Sometimes a partner might suggest giving the other a foot massage, sometimes they might desire simply to lie down and touch one another intimately or engage in sexual fantasy role play. If they can find a way to say what they want, and preserve open communication, then their intimate lives, whatever they are, will be happier.

In this context, putting in place a time-out is a really positive thing. A safe word, or a call for a stop that is immediately understood and respected, allows you and your intimate partner to take responsibility for yourselves and so allows more freedom of exploration both physically and emotionally. It is a positive part of sexual play to be encouraged from the time of teenagers' sexual awakening.

Continuing to negotiate actively throughout all the ages and stages of your life is the key. I've increasingly come to understand that our intimate needs should be talked about without too much expectation but with absolute openness—and with an acceptance that what you want at different moments of your life will change. Linsey Blair likens it to eating. You decide to eat and what to eat, depending on how hungry you are, and what kind of food you feel like having. Maybe you want a piece of toast. Or perhaps you desire a three-course meal. Perhaps you want something exotic and unusual, or something plain and comforting. You don't ever walk into a restaurant and order something you don't want to eat; you are unlikely to eat until you feel sick. You balance your needs and your desires with different and varying kinds of food.

She suggests that couples regard intimacy as a kind of tapas menu. You might try one or two things and leave it at that. You might experiment with a dish you haven't eaten before. But you order in bite-sized chunks; you don't just think every sexual encounter has to be a three-course meal leading to penetration and orgasm. Sometimes doing small things every day is more intimate than a three-course extravaganza once every three months.

You can lie down and stroke each other for 15 minutes and then have a hug. You can have a bath together. You can go for a walk and hold hands or stand in the night under the stars. It is for everyone to find out what suits them. But if you keep cultivating intimate gestures, nurturing your intimate connection, when you do come to "eat a three-course meal," then the sparks can fly as you are more in tune with each other!

Sometimes by being honest with a partner, you may find that your hopes and desires and the ways you wish to live your life develop and change. It is important in our intimate relationships not to hold each other too close—to allow a little space for electricity between us. Living together is difficult for a lot of people; long-term intimacy can be a challenge. In allowing someone space, you may drift apart and find you are on different paths. Having one intimate partner for a long time is not for everyone. Freedom is a part of openness, and sometimes the most loving gift you can give to a partner is to let them go if that is what is required. It takes courage and true unconditional love to recognize when a relationship has run its course and to allow each of you to move on.

The intention to strive for open communication and to engage in a beautiful, intimate, sexual, ever-evolving relationship with a loved one, or loved ones, is a challenging part of who we are as human beings. To listen to yourself and really know what you are feeling in the moment in yourself, and in relation to your partner, is hard. Finding the right time to communicate also takes negotiation and good timing within a busy world full of pressures.

This may only be achieved in moments, but the intention to be in this place with someone else is the important thing. But by staying present we can be truly intimate with ourselves, and so with our partners, and hopefully go on to have lives that are more fulfilled in every aspect.

HOW TO ASK

It can be hard to know exactly what we want in our intimate relationships, and I hope that what we've explored so far reassures you that this is part of a life-long journey of connection with ourselves and our partners. Even when we do know what we want, it can feel challenging to know how to ask for it!

In this exercise, I invite you to create a safe space with your partner in which you can both share with open hearts and minds. There is nothing to judge: this is an opportunity to give and receive the suggestions, and to sit with them together.

- First, agree in advance a time with your partner when you can feel confident you'll be undisturbed. Explain that you would like to share this moment with them, sharing your reflections and inviting them to share theirs.

- If sitting opposite your partner feels a bit too intense, another really good way you could create a space for this conversation is to go on a walk together somewhere calm and quiet, such as in nature, where you can talk as you walk.

- In a quiet space, be seated facing each other, so that you can enjoy the intimate experience of eye contact.

- Decide who will speak first. You might agree to spend two minutes each, and during this time for the receiver to focus on listening, without judgment or interruption.

- Share your desires with your partner in the level of detail that feels good to you. You might wish to ask for something specific that you would like to incorporate into your intimate life, such as a sexual position, but you may also wish to ask for something more general— for example, to renew the focus on your intimacy—or for something that isn't sexual. For example, you might be asking to spend more time together, to enjoy more nonsexual physical contact such as hugging or holding hands. You can ask for anything here, in the knowledge that you are free from judgment.

- When you speak about your desires, try to speak from a positive space, rather than one of criticism of your partner. For example, rather than saying, "You don't do this," you might say, "I'd love to do more of that." I invite you to tell your partner why what you are asking for might feel good to you.

- Swap roles. Now take the opportunity to listen to your partner for their two minutes. Once again, there is no need to respond or make a judgment. Instead, allow yourself to really listen to what is being shared, acknowledging this shared place of safety you have created together.

- After you have both spoken, take a minute of silence to absorb what you have both expressed. Notice how it felt for you to share your desire. Also notice how it felt to receive a desire from your partner, and what this might be bringing to your mind.

> » Do you feel excited?

> » Do you feel inspired?

> » Do you feel nervous?

> » Do you have further questions?

> » How does this exchange feel in your body?

- Next, the first speaker invites the first listener to respond. You might start by asking, "How did it feel to hear me say that?" Be curious and open as you embark on this discussion once you have listened to their answer, remembering this is not about judgment but about engaging with the way each of you feel. If something makes you uncomfortable or you feel it might take you beyond your boundaries, tell your partner how you feel: this is an opportunity for you to both understand each other more deeply.

- Swap roles, so that the second speaker can ask the second listener how they received their desires. Once again, speak from a place of kindness and curiosity.

- Once you have explored both roles, take a moment to consider together what might come next. What would you like to explore together, and how might you bring it into your shared intimate lives? Can you make a commitment to trying some of these new things together, in a way that feels safe and comfortable for you both?

- Remember, this is a journey, not a destination. Don't feel the pressure to transform everything about your intimate life from a single experience of this exercise. Instead, revisit it regularly, allowing you and your partner the opportunity to share what might be changing and evolving for you, keeping an open exploration of your shared intimacy.

CHAPTER ELEVEN

FINDING THE ENCHANTRESS

AND INTIMACY INTO OUR OLDER YEARS

The actress Greta Scacchi was interviewed in 2023 about her huge fame in the 1980s, when she starred in films such as *Heat and Dust* and *White Mischief.* "It was very clear to me even then that I was always being invited to play a male fantasy," she said. "I had to work very hard to punch some integrity into the idea of being a woman when I was placed inside that male gaze."

Noting that things had changed a lot over her 40-year career, and that there were many more female directors working, she added: "But the way older women get portrayed is often still very odd. I call it the gray wig in the wardrobe problem . . . But many women don't look gray-wigged . . . Where are the glamorous—or even not glamorous—representations of today's older women? Where are the women who went through women's lib? Flower power? The punk chicks? Just because we're playing people over 60, we shouldn't be playing outdated preconceptions of what we are."[1]

I couldn't have put it better myself. It's one of the instances where film is slow in reflecting a broader change in society where women—and men as well—see 50 as a halfway staging post in their lives rather than as a step closer to retirement. When I was young, grannies looked really old to me, and they had gray, tightly permed hair. Retirees were people waiting to die, rather than a group just beginning a new phase of their lives.

Now, thanks to improvements in medicine and fitness, reaching the official retirement age might simply mean that you've got a significant chunk of your life left. This has implications for almost everything, including intimacy. Yet the trajectory of our lives that we most often see reflected at us still shows significant differences between views of men and views of women.

Men are depicted as silver foxes, rugged, lined, and sexy. They are figures of power, influence, and attraction. Women get to their 40s and then suddenly, mainly, become invisible until they reappear as grannies. As actress Andie MacDowell remarked: "I still think there is this concept that men are handsome as they age, and women are not. I think these outdated terms need to be thought through. I would like to see more acting roles that show women aging in all their power and natural beauty; I'd like to visually see it in advertising, films, and television. Men get to age, and women need to be able to age as well. That's it in a nutshell . . . I don't want to have to pretend to be what I'm not."[2]

As I've noted earlier, our culture seems to be pushing back. Women are asserting their right to be seen and understood as vibrant older people in the same way as men. Nowhere is this more obvious than in the changing attitudes to menopause that have been led by a new generation of female campaigners, who grew up in the 1960s and are simply not prepared to let this time in women's lives be treated as something shameful that has to be endured in silence.

At the time I was writing this book, the National Health Service estimated that there were around 13 million people in the UK who were perimenopausal or menopausal, which is equivalent to a third of the entire UK female population.[3] The wide range of physical and psychological symptoms of this entirely natural change in the body can last for several years and includes hot flushes, short-term memory loss, extreme anxiety, mood swings, night sweats, and difficulty sleeping. Yet, until very recently, such symptoms were either ignored or ridiculed.

Prominent women, such as the TV presenters Davina McCall and Mariella Frostrup in the UK, have led the way for women to talk about menopause more openly, campaigning for a recognition that it is a life-changing moment that requires support and understanding in the workplace and in the home.

In the US, the actor Naomi Watts took on the role of chair of Menopause Mandate, the US counterpart of Frostrup's UK organization. Based on their own experiences of feeling like strangers to themselves when they hit this time in their lives, all of these women have campaigned for hormone replacement therapies (HRT) to be more widely available and better understood, and for more support and understanding to be given to women going through a time of transition where, according to the British Menopause

Society, more than 75 percent of women experience menopausal symptoms, with a quarter describing their symptoms as severe. A third of these women experience long-term symptoms, which may last as much as seven years or more.[4]

McCall said she felt she had become an accidental activist. "You don't want to make a fuss because you're embarrassed . . . You feel like perhaps an older stateswoman in the business will not be valued and that the menopause will be aging. So, you don't tell people that you're struggling. And then, you think you're in fear of your job but then you don't get any support. And then the worst thing happens: you really do feel like you can't do it anymore and then you leave."[5]

It's exciting that in this day and age, we are finally lifting the lid off the effects of menopause and that as women, we are giving ourselves permission to be more vocal about what we are going through without facing criticism. In this context, how we view women in their middle and older years starts to change because women can acknowledge the aging process within their bodies without being penalized for it in the workplace or without struggling on in silence in their intimate lives, even though their needs may have altered.

This is one reason that Linsey Blair talks about expanding the definition of intimacy and of sex. There is no doubt that penetration-focused intimacy is often problematic for older women and those undergoing menopause, because the vaginal walls thin and penetrative intercourse becomes painful. Advocates such as Frostrup suggest that HRT provides an answer to this, and new developments in HRT, including the use of bioidentical hormone replacement therapy, are supporting many women. Estrogen pessaries may also be useful in making intercourse more enjoyable. These are certainly positive options to offer, as are other ways to support you through the menopause. Supplements, such as magnesium and sage leaf, can be a very effective and inexpensive method of improving your physical and mental health.[6] Homeopathic remedies are another resource for support through this time in life, along with considering a diet and fitness plan.

In this, as in so many things, as a pioneer of exercise at all stages of life, actor and activist Jane Fonda continues to inspire in her late 80s. "I credit exercise with having a good life," she said as she launched a new series of workouts for Supernatural, a virtual reality fitness platform. "When you're younger, working out is a choice. When you're older, working out is an absolute necessity. It makes all the difference in the world whether you'll be able to get in and out of a car, carry your own luggage, play with your grandkids, have a life. If you don't keep moving when you're over 50, you're going to lose your life." She's very funny about it. "The mantra becomes slower. It's kind of like sex—slower." But she is also a shining example of the way in which embracing a shift in life that is natural and normal and supporting yourself in different ways can help you to journey into a transition into the postmenopausal and older years.[7]

In general, it's important that doctors who are dealing with women who are perimenopausal and menopausal are better educated about the options they can offer. One trend which campaigners have highlighted is the tendency to over-prescribe antidepressants to women reporting with perimenopausal symptoms. Again, this may help some women, but it is worrying that prescription drugs and medical treatment are offered as a quick fix for a problem that is, after all, an entirely natural occurrence.

I always think it is a beautiful thing that a female baby in her mother's womb contains all the eggs that she will produce in her reproductive life. Effectively, if a woman gives birth to a girl, she is giving birth to the seed of her own grandchildren. Once those ova are used, that is it! That's one reason menopause is such a sharp process. Ovulation ends and hormone production drops over a relatively short period of time. It is really the end of something.

The male menopause—or the andropause, as it is sometimes known—is a different and much more gradual process. Indeed, some health experts think that using the term to describe symptoms, which include mood swings, a general lack of enthusiasm and energy, poor concentration and short-term memory, in men in their late 40s to early 50s is misleading because, as the NHS says, it suggests that the symptoms are the result of a sudden drop in testosterone in middle age similar to the female menopause.

Men continue to produce sperm throughout their lives; that's why men in their 80s can still father children. Although testosterone levels do fall as men age, it drops around 1 percent a year and is unlikely to cause any problems in itself. A different condition—a testosterone deficiency known as late-onset hypogonadism—may cause some of the symptoms but, in many cases, they are nothing to do with hormones and will be treated differently. Recommendations on testosterone therapy for men with age-related low testosterone vary.[8]

What is clear, however, is that all these feelings, physical and emotional, produce a need to see intimacy in new ways. In the past decade, Linsey Blair has encountered a new phenomenon where straight women leave their husbands and establish a relationship with another woman. "I don't know how to explain it, but it is to do with the fact that women are really changing. Historically, as they grew older and were post-fertility, they didn't live that long. But where we now are, post-childbirth and post-fertility, penetrative sex makes no sense and women perhaps just do not desire the sex they were having anymore. They want something different.

Blair continues, "When you've got maybe 30 years of your life left, and your children have grown up and moved away, you have to decide whether you want to be with this particular partner. Perhaps the qualities that originally attracted you to them are not so strong anymore. You've changed. Perhaps women don't want to be in the caregiver's role anymore, they want more equal sharing of household duties. They want something that feels equal, different, softer. And they want someone to chat to.

"It is a time when couples just have to really reassess, look at each other and decide again. A lot of women decide no. Interestingly, the men less so. They are a lot happier than the women. It's a massive shift for women to say, I want to look after me now, stop being a caregiver and move on."

Even without making so radical a decision, it is clear that menopause is a crossroad of immense change and possibility. It is a time when women have gathered a full life of experience, skills, and wisdom and yet are still full of vitality and energy. They have more space in life, to give to themselves, have a career, and give back to society. If they are lucky their children are in their early 20s and no longer needing them for the intense caregiving that they did in their childhood years. Their parents are hopefully still healthy enough to have their own autonomy in their older years. In this place, people have a possible 20-year window where they can really question and conduct their lives in a way that allows them to express themselves as they weren't able to do previously.

A lot of people find themselves freer than at any point since their teenage years, yet with a bit more money to spend and a little more knowledge at their backs.

In terms of intimacy, from the moment they begin to menstruate, women's sexual lives are governed by either the need to prevent a pregnancy or by the desire to get pregnant. It's no wonder that this period of huge physical and psychological change offers new possibilities for established relationships and perhaps sets different parameters for establishing new ones. What this indicates is that keeping our intimate lives alive isn't only about maintaining a physical sexual life together, but also about talking, about finding space to be with someone and continue to grow and change alongside them. It suggests that for women, in particular, this is a stage of their lives to be relished.

There's a simplified archetypal definition of the ages of women that runs maiden, mother, crone. But increased longevity in many cultures means that women don't simply tip from being a mother to being an old woman. New thinking suggests that this misses out one of the most important stages: woman as an enchantress. This is the age between mother and crone: a woman who, postmenopausal, is embracing her life; a woman at her blossoming best, with new energy and power. She is through her child-rearing years and has no thought of pregnancy. The cycles of hormones have ended—and she is in a position where she can explore and engage with the world on her own terms!

With regards to the seasons, a young person is in the spring of their life, the child rearer in the summer, and this enchantress phase takes place during the autumn, before the winter of old age. The enchantress can relax into intimacy and sexual encounters purely for pleasure. There is nothing else other than who you are with yourself, with your partner, and with the connection that you have with each other. It is pure joy.

In the second series of *Fleabag* by Phoebe Waller-Bridge, a series which does so much to talk honestly and openly about women's intimate and emotional lives, there's a scene in which the heroine meets a successful businesswoman called Belinda (played by Kristin Scott Thomas) at an awards ceremony. As a writer, Waller-Bridge gives the character an extraordinary monologue about what it is to be a woman.

"Women are built with pain built in," Belinda says. "It's our physical destiny: period pains, sore boobs, childbirth, you know. We carry it within ourselves throughout our lives; men don't. They have to seek it out, they invent all these gods and demons and things just so they can feel guilty about things, which is something we do very well on our own. And then they create wars so they can feel things and touch each other and when there aren't any wars, they can play rugby.

"We have it all going on in here, inside, we have pain on

a cycle for years and years and years and then just when you feel you are making peace with it all, what happens? The menopause comes, the fucking menopause comes, and it is the most wonderful fucking thing in the world. And yes, your entire pelvic floor crumbles and you get fucking hot and no one cares, but then you're free, no longer a slave, no longer a machine with parts. You're just a person . . . It is horrendous. But then it's magnificent. Something to look forward to."[9]

I love that so much. It's the kind of speech that seems to sum up what so many women have felt, are feeling, and go on feeling. It makes you want to shout with joy. Perfectly delivered, with precision timing and poise by Scott Thomas, it is a recognition of all the ways in which women suffer— and a celebration of the time of their lives when women truly have a chance to become the enchantress, to be their own wild selves.

This might show itself in all kinds of ways, by pushing on further in careers, by exercising more, by taking up yoga or going to the gym, by enjoying friendships with new people, by traveling and going on adventures to far-flung places, by pushing boundaries in all directions with the confidence and wisdom of age but also with the freedom from the responsibility of the child-rearing years.

It's in this context that they can reshape their intimate lives. One consideration of the menopause years for couples who live with each other is that they end up in separate bedrooms. Once people are separated in this way, it can become more difficult to initiate intimacy because people just aren't spending as much time together in an intimate setting anymore. Equally, with the hormonal surges of the menstrual cycle out of the way, it might be that women don't have the same flow of sexual arousal, that they feel more neutral about intimate activity. Your longing for the next intimate encounter will be based on your memory of the last; if that memory was unpleasant or painful, then it is less likely to make you want to initiate sexual activity.

Communication, as ever, is the solution to these hurdles. If you're in separate rooms, there has to be much more chatting around sex—an invitation perhaps from one person to the other to share a bed at the same time. And then, perhaps, you'll leave. Perhaps you will have oral sex or share some other form of arousal. Perhaps in this period, you won't have more than a hug. But you will be together and will be intimate with one another. For some people, emotional intimacy is more important than having an orgasm; others will value physical stimulation more; for others, the introduction of vibrators and lubrication might now be part of the intimate play. But by scheduling the time together and talking about what each other wants, you have a chance of keeping your intimate life alive. The script needs to change. You can't simply assume that the person you are with will still want the same thing they always have wanted; they might want something different, and the only way to discover that is to talk about it, honestly and openly.

A survey published in the British medical magazine *The Lancet* reported that 86 percent of men and 60 percent of women aged 60–69 said they were sexually active, falling to 59 percent of men and 34 percent of women aged 70–79.[10] While there were physical challenges to achieving a satisfying sex life, such as vaginal changes during menopause, erectile dysfunction, or mobility issues,

Miranda Christophers, a sex and relationship expert for the online menopause platform Issviva, emphasizes the health benefits, in terms of building self-esteem, the release of chemicals that boost the immune system and the lowering of stress. She notes that many older people are now consulting therapists to discover ways of maintaining sexual relationships—and starting new ones.[11]

Difficulties arise because societal attitudes shift so slowly. Just as Scacchi resists the gray wig, so we need to learn not to imagine our older people as some kind of sexless blob, fading into grayness. Most people need intimacy—which may or may not lead to sexual activity—as long as they live. In August 2022, social workers Shirley Ayres and Mervyn Eastman, members of the Sexual Intimacy in Later Life UK Forum, published what they called "a provocation paper" called "Sex, Intimacy and Sexual Wellbeing in Later Life" in which they invited various contributions on the theme. Sharron Hinchliff, professor of psychology and health in the division of nursing and midwifery at Sheffield University, notes that although there has been a significant shift in the way that the sexuality of older adults is now viewed in Western societies, the stereotype of older people as frail, sick, and in decline is still dominant. "Not all stereotypes are damaging," she writes. "But the stereotype of a sexless older age can be. It can prevent open and honest conversation about sexual health and well-being, thereby perpetuating myths and misunderstandings." She goes on to argue that, "One way to put aging and sexual health and well-being on the health and social care agenda is to take a rights-based approach. Sexual rights are human rights as applied to sexuality."[12]

I feel this is a positive approach. Supporting our elders in their intimate needs and desires really starts with open communication, as I've shared throughout this book, beginning with conversations between the couples themselves to negotiate their wants and desires. It also requires open conversations between older people and their grown-up children. This can be challenging. Invariably, no one wants to think about their parents having sex, let alone their grandparents. However, it is important to normalize these conversations so this area of life can be supported.

If one or other of your parents goes into a retirement home, it is important that this aspect of who they are and how they require to be supported in their intimate and sexual needs is given as much focus and attention as what they like to eat and what activities and exercise they enjoy. Likewise, it is important that the policies in the homes support sexual health. As Dr. Jane Youell states in the section of the report *Sexuality in Residential and Nursing Homes*, "when Jack masturbates at bath time this might be because that is the only time he has access to his own naked body (some private alone time in his room without a pad on might help). Or that Joanie might like access to a sex toy because she misses sex with her late husband."[13]

This type of understanding can only grow if there are policies in residential and social care that normalize the support of sexual and intimate needs. If those polices are not in place, then it affects people's behavior by preventing them from seeking help should they have a sexual issue. "It can have serious consequences and put an end to a much-longed-for sex life," Hinchliff says. Within the LGBTQ+

community, the consequences can include pushing individuals back into the closet by failing to deal with an atmosphere of secrecy and shame.

For so many people, this time of life can deepen and strengthen their bonds of intimacy. It is also true, however, that in continuing to be curious and to change and alter definitions of what they want from their relationships, some couples discover that they are journeying along different paths and that they can no longer stay together. As discussed, this has led to the phenomenon of the "gray divorce."

An analysis of divorce data from 1990 to 2021 released in July 2023 by Bowling Green State University's National Center for Family and Marriage Research in the US found that divorce rates for those aged 45 and over rose during that period, while rates dropped for those younger than 45. The most significant increase was among people aged 65 and over, which tripled in those 11 years. Researchers on the study argued that these rising divorce rates among "boomers," or people born between 1946 and 1964, weren't because their relationships were more conflicted than those in other age groups. Instead, they put the increase down to the fact that society is now more tolerant of divorce, and women have become more financially and emotionally independent.[14]

Working and researching in film and TV, looking at people's changing lives, I feel these shifts all around me. Gradually we are seeing older women in all their power and beauty. *Nomadland,* which won the best picture Oscar in 2021, starred the ultimate "eldress" Frances McDormand and concentrated on the resonance of her character's life, including her friendships and her attractions. *Everything*

Everywhere All at Once, which won best picture in 2023, turned its gaze firmly on the apparently ordinary life of a middle-aged woman in the shape of Michelle Yeoh, whose character in the course of the film was allowed, in various time slips, to show herself in every possibility— downtrodden launderette owner, mother, warrior, and enchantress.

It's not just the Oscar winners who are changing the focus. In a similar way, Katharine Hardman, who was intimacy coordinator on *The Great,* the brilliant counter-historical series starring Elle Fanning as Catherine the Great of Russia, noted how wonderful it was to work with Ninette Finch, an actress in her 80s, and choreograph a screen kiss with a much younger man. "We were just like, this is brilliant, this should be happening all the time."[15] When it does, it's so empowering—and not just for straight women. In the third episode of *The Last of Us,* Nick Offerman and Murray Bartlett played Bill and Frank, a couple of middle-aged men. It was directed by Peter Hoar, who also directed *It's a Sin*—and it was so overwhelmingly moving that after watching it, I contacted him to congratulate him on such a positive depiction of older people in a physically affectionate relationship.[16]

I felt the same when, in 2021, the relationships charity Relate commissioned the photographer Rankin to take a series of portraits of older people, to celebrate intimacy in the later years. I helped with the campaign, which featured five real-life couples and one woman in sensual poses, by checking to make sure everyone was comfortable and happy with the way that they were photographed and filmed. It was a wonderful event to be part of because their connection with their own bodies (wrinkles, gray hair, and all) was so intense that it really communicated the joy of our relationships as we reach our 70s and beyond. Launching the campaign, Rankin said: "The simple fact is, we all need intimacy now more than ever—and age really is just a number. The greatness of love and affection—the very things we can't stop writing books, films and pop songs about—doesn't need to change . . ."[17]

Faced with statistics that showed sex and intimacy among people over 65 years of age was never or rarely represented in the media, and that the majority (60 percent) of older people weren't comfortable talking openly about it, the campaign offered such a positive and inspiring experience of intimacy in our later years.[18] The film and photographs featured Andrew and Mark, who had been together for 31 years; Chrissie, who had had a double mastectomy, with her partner Roger; and Daphne and Arthur, who still hold hands when they go for a walk.

The comments that accompanied the images were revealing. Mark, who was 61, and 67-year-old Andrew talked about the fact that they got more experimental in intimacy as they got older. "You've got to mix it up . . . it might be infrequent, but the older you get, the better you get at it." Chrissie, 71, and her 81-year-old partner Roger admitted that there had been challenges to having sex when they were older—mainly to do with health and being uncomfortable after surgery—but asserted that "the intimacy, the love that a couple share often shines through." They added: "A lot of people think older people are past it. That they don't have the inner feelings of love and touch that you have when you are younger, but in fact it has surprised us both that you do maintain exactly those same feelings and you want to touch each other."

Research underlines the truth of these observations, showing that although the frequency of sexual activity may naturally decrease as people get older, the quality and pleasure often increases as people have a more positive attitude to their bodies and more confidence about stating their needs and exploring ways of being intimate that will help them overcome any physical challenges.

The photographs gave such a positive image of older bodies, both queer and straight, it felt revelatory and in emphasizing the qualities of touch and physical contact, they emphasized the happiness that intimacy can bring. Working on them reminded me of seeing Pina Bausch's radical dance work "Kontakthof," set in a dance hall, where couples come together to dance and explore sexual relationships, in all their joy and pain.

At one point, Bausch set the work (originally made for her own company, Tanztheater Wuppertal) on two separate companies of amateur performers: one group were over 60, the other were teenagers of 16 and 17. I saw the performance of the older cast with my mother, and the younger cast with my teenage daughter. We tend to think of sexiness and flirtatiousness as the domain of the young; we revere and focus on the beauty of youth, and treat older people as invisible, with no desire, sensuality, or sexuality. Yet those performances upended that idea.

The show opens with the dancers coming forward one at a time to stare into an unseen mirror, examining their bodies, preening, as they lift their breasts, check their profile, examine their teeth. What struck me was it was the older people who were actually in their bodies, who exuded desire and sexiness, who embodied all the frisson of joy in the intimate play of relationships. The young people were beautiful, of course, but they didn't know how to wear their stylish dresses or how to present themselves. They were timid and awkward as they stepped forward with all the expectation and hope of finding a partner.

Dancing exactly the same steps, it was the older people who had that sense of life in their bodies. They understood their power and had a confidence that made them utterly gorgeous. It was a reminder of the fact that it is how we feel that makes us beautiful and sexy, not how we look.

It's a joy to remember that there's so much to be experienced later in our lives. I was reminded of this when I first encountered shamanic Moon Cycles, which offer a very different way of thinking about the beautiful and full cycle of our long lives. According to Thunder Strikes and Jan Orsi, ancient shamanic cultures use "the teachings of the Star Maidens Circle [to] describe our life experiences in the Moon Cycles . . . We journey from infancy to our elder years in cycles of twenty-seven years."[19] They describe the Moon Cycle phases as follows:

The Child Moon runs from birth to the age of 27, years which "are spent developing your personality and creating your mythology and stories about who you are."

The Adolescent Moon, from age 27 to 54, "is the time for accomplishing goals, achieving success, stability and even abundance."

The Adult Moon, from 54 to 81, is where you reap the harvest of your life experience. "At this point, you will either enter your mature years with ease, grace and a sense of fulfillment, or become set in your belief systems and unwilling to make changes. These years offer the opportunity to devote more time and energy to personal growth, perhaps even to seek adventure and further explore the unknown in spiritual development."

The Elder Moon, from 81 onward "is the moon you enter with wisdom and honor for the legacy you have created, or you can end with regrets and resignation waiting for death to come. Few people reach this age today with vitality and eagerness to explore the years ahead, yet these can be the years rich with illuminations and enlightening experiences."

That's always felt an entirely convincing trajectory of life to me—and it becomes more and more relevant as people live so much longer. I had a sense I was playing at being an adult until I reached around 50 when I then had some sense of who I was and what I was doing. I look forward to becoming an elder, when my knowledge will deepen still further.

As we are living longer, then the invitation is to stay open and vital to what life has to offer to sustain and develop our intimate and loving relationships well into our older age.

CONCLUSION

The hero or heroine's journey is one of the archetypal structures for storytelling and theater. It takes an arc where a person, safe at home, feels the need to embark on an exploration or an adventure. They set out with high hopes but doubt themselves as they get further away from what is comfortable and known. They're tempted to return to safety. But they keep going, battling adversity, until they realize that to turn back would be as treacherous as going forward.

Once they are truly on the path, meeting helpers or mentors along the way, experiencing challenges and temptations, they reach a point where they can do nothing except descend into the abyss, where they meet the demon that they must slay, which is very often a part of themselves. After they have faced their greatest fears by killing the demon, the demon gives them a gift to bring back. They set out on their return journey, having transformed, knowing themselves in a different and deeper way than before and bringing that gift back to their loved ones.

It is the basis for stories from *The Odyssey* to *The Lion King*. *Star Wars* owes it a debt too. So does *The Last of Us*.

One of the reasons it is so pervasive is that this mythic structure helps us make sense of the challenges of our lives, of learning and changing under the pressure of experience. However, while the hero or heroine's journey is as old as storytelling itself, sometimes we need to refresh our scripts. My hope is that this book will help you rewrite the script so that you can find connection with yourselves and others at every stage of your life.

When we commit to telling our own stories on our own terms, this honest communication is what defines true intimacy, and it's what also drives the hero/heroine's journey. My career and this book have had elements of that journey. It is said that you teach best what you most need to learn. In the exploration and research I have gathered working as an intimacy practitioner, and in speaking with experts such as Linsey Blair, Dr. Siobhán O'Higgins, and Dr. Orna Guralnik, I feel I have been profoundly educated, and my attitude toward my own sexuality and sensuality has been enriched. I have been able to take that learning into my loving relationships.

I feel I have two starting points. Since I was a child, the pleasure of moving, of expressing my emotions and feelings through the physicality of music, movement, and dance, has given me joy—a joy I want to share. My place of challenge is the effect of my Catholic upbringing, where anything to do with intimacy and sex was shrouded in a veil of secrecy, ignorance, shame, and guilt.

Bridging the gap between those two things set me on the path of choreographing intimacy professionally. The idea of open communication, agreement and consent, choreography, and closure in the depiction of intimacy in the arts has also allowed me to find a way to celebrate who we are as human beings in our intimate lives. Researching this book, I feel I have reached a more expansive understanding of how intimacy can be deepened if we continue to be honest with ourselves and with each other in investigating our feelings and desires, and how we can express our sensuality and sexuality with ourselves and our loved ones.

The different kinds of intimacy we develop with our partners, our children, and our friends are the core of human connection. They take different forms: our sexual energy is our life force that can culminate in the miracle of the creation of a new life; our relationships with our children nourish and nurture that life; our relationships with our friends enrich it. Lacking the ability to forge intimate relationships can damage us, cutting us off from pleasure, from our creative energy, from our ability to express ourselves.

In each sphere of intimacy, the willingness to be open and honest is everything. The underlying theme of this book, my work, and my life is the need for open communication and transparency. There is no substitute for it, and it's almost impossible to move forward without it. I feel my own trajectory, from a naïve teenager to an intimacy coordinator who can use direct language that doesn't obscure anything and who can help build a clearer and more truthful picture of intimacy onscreen, is in some ways a reflection of how things are changing.

If we can't talk about our intimate relations, then we have little hope of improving them. This extends through every stage of life. If we improve our sex education, we can support every young person to understand the true meaning of active consent, so they will not ever think no means yes, or that reluctance is feigned.

Through this work, we can encourage everyone to listen to themselves and to have the language to treat one another with respect and negotiate intimate relations in calm and present ways. I hope this book has helped to lift the lid on the damage of ignorance and repression, and is a call to arms to develop a way of viewing intimacy that is easily accessible and a viable alternative to the go-to of pornography, helping people journey through their sexual awakening in a way that allows them to celebrate who they are, respect their boundaries and the boundaries of others, and take this joy for life and pleasure into their sexual explorations and relationships.

When women are empowered, it also frees our boys and men to stand in their power, offering their strength of masculinity in service—be it in the work they do, in their intimate relationships, and as fathers in the home. I wonder whether older men, who discover the value of emotional closeness and who learn to talk to their partners about their needs, might inspire young boys and men who are still so strongly bound up in old-fashioned definitions of masculinity and scared to open up and explore relationships.

Keeping communication open can be challenging. But it is what I am advocating for. Underlying this entire book is my sense that if we can base all our intimate relationships—be they sexual or nonsexual—on respect, communication, and openness, then we are setting a template for how our society and our communities can be more measured and more tolerant. We can begin to write a different hero or heroine's journey, one that faces challenges but emerges with new stories to tell.

Some of those stories will be reflected on our screens and our stages, telling different tales about who we are now. But others, importantly, will be embodied in our lives and the ways we choose to live in our communities and with the people we love.

Let me go back to the questions I asked at the very start of this book, the ones that form the basis of all our intimate relationships. *Who am I? What do I need? Where am I going? What are my desires? What are my fantasies?* They are questions we need to ask ourselves and our partners. *Who are they? What do they need? Where are they going? What are their desires and fantasies?*

They are questions that will have different answers at different points in our lives, but if we keep asking them, keep rewriting the scripts of our own journey, then our intimate lives will deepen and expand. I hope this book brings a gift to you, the reader, and offers you a field guide to understanding your own intimate life and relationships.

ACKNOWLEDGMENTS

I'm so grateful to have been given the opportunity to share my practice. In developing and working with the Intimacy on Set Guidelines, I have been inspired and nurtured by so many people, without whom this contribution to the industry would not exist in its current form.

I have such gratitude for Katie Rose for supporting me since 2014 while I developed these ideas in a devised piece, *Does My Sex Offend You?*, and for her invaluable counsel ever since.

I am grateful to Meredith Dufton, who invited me to teach the work at Mountview Academy of Theatre Arts in April of 2015, and who was instrumental in honing the guidelines. Meredith had the insight, in exercising her duty of care to her students, to seriously question the creation of intimate content. Thank you also to Vanessa Ewan of the Royal Central School of Speech & Drama, for her generous support in developing this practice. In particular, chapter nine of *Actor Movement: Expression of the Physical Being*

(Bloomsbury Methuen Drama, 2015) provided a springboard to further exploration.

My profound and heartfelt thanks goes also to Fiona Gillies, my mentor on a scheme run by Women in Film and Television in early 2018 as I was taking my first tentative steps on set as an intimacy coordinator, and for her continued guidance in the development of the Intimacy on Set Practitioner training. Her support in unpacking the challenges and developing robust processes and protocols has been invaluable.

Thank you to each and every intimacy practitioner student who has joined me at Intimacy on Set. I have learned so much from the times when the work has been successful and joyous, and I've learned even more when it has been challenging and confronting. The process of reflection and development is ongoing, and I'm thankful to everybody who has developed the work with me, right through to those who are working with me now and will be into the future.

I feel privileged to have had the opportunity to support so many incredible productions. I thank the writers, producers, directors, actors, costume designers, makeup, cinematographers, and crew. You have all been my teachers. Special thanks to Michaela Cole, whose BAFTA acceptance speech in 2021 highlighted the importance of intimacy coordinators in the industry.

I want to thank everyone at Penguin: to Hana Teraie-Wood for seeing me and understanding my practice and the possibility of what I had to share. Thank you to Robyn Drury, Emily Martin, Whitney Frick, and Sam Zukergood for your unwavering support. As they say, the art of writing is the art of rewriting! I am honored to be a

Penguin author; it is a wonderful privilege to be in such great company.

Thank you to my literary agent, Chris Wellbelove, for his gentle guidance and care throughout the process of writing this book.

I am a dancer and a mover. As a dyslexic person, putting my inspiration into the written word is a place of challenge. So, I am incredibly grateful to Sarah Crompton for supporting me with her wonderful writing skills, her in-depth knowledge of movement and dance, and her endless patience.

Finally, I could not have done any of this without my family. You are my bedrock, my support, my sounding board, and have literally kept my body and soul alive as I've been putting together this book. With so much love and gratitude, thank you to my partner, Russell, and my children, Zac and Zoe.

APPENDICES

INTIMACY ON SET GUIDELINES

BEST PRACTICE WHEN WORKING WITH INTIMACY,
SIMULATED SEX SCENES, AND NUDITY

1. Producers to identify whether a production may include
   scenes of intimacy and sexual content as part of the risk
   assessment; ensure that relevant departments are
   informed and necessary measures put in place:

   a. Put in place wardrobe—appropriate covering for
      genitalia.
   b. Crew required for a closed set.
   c. Consideration of, and budget for, an Intimacy
      Coordinator.

2. No initial auditions or screen tests are to include sex
   scenes or to involve nudity. Where, in exceptional
   circumstances, nudity or semi-nudity is required in a
   recall, the actor must be informed in advance and be
   provided with the script. All material recorded must be
   protected and be destroyed once the role has been
   cast.

a. The actor to sign a written agreement with the Casting Director that any recording of a nude or semi-nude audition will be confidential.

b. The actor may be asked to audition in specific clothing (e.g., swimwear) required for a commercial but will be informed in advance.

c. If an actor is nude or semi-nude in a recall, they may bring a support person to be with them throughout the shoot.

d. The only other people allowed to be present in the audition room will be the Casting Director and/or Director/Producer, and the Reader.

3. At point of contract all scenes involving nudity, intimacy, or simulated sex to be discussed with the actor and their representative/agent, so that agreement is made with full disclosure.

a. The standard Equity contract for screen productions allows the actor to agree, or disagree, to performing nude and to performing simulated sex and to choose the type of nudity the actor is willing to do (e.g., buttocks only, or full frontal).

b. Actors sometimes accept a role in which their character will be semi-nude, only to find later that additional scenes have been written into the script which include full-frontal nudity and simulated sex. Actors should not sign a contract for full-frontal nudity and simulated sex if only prepared to go semi-nude.

4. Directors to plainly describe and discuss with the relevant actors all scenes involving intimacy, simulated

sex, and nudity at the appropriate times in the creative process:
- a. before signing the contract;
- b. throughout the rehearsal process;
- c. and into performance.

5. Agreement and consent by the actor, and actors' representative, to be given each and every time when working with intimacy, simulated sex scenes, and nudity.

6. Establish boundaries around areas of concern, including an agreed strategy to halt the action where necessary, in rehearsals and filming on set, such as "time out."

7. When sculpting intimacy or a simulated sex scene, for the actor and Director, or the actor and Director in conjunction with an Intimacy Coordinator, to follow the Intimacy on Set Guidelines as standard practice.
- a. Always have a third party present, keeping the work professional, not private.
- b. Identify the blocking of the scene.
- c. Agree areas of physical touch.
- d. Sculpt the physical actions using plain words.
- e. Separately identify the emotional content of the scene.
- f. Integrate the physical actions and emotional content, creating a seamless intimate scene.

8. Onstage, when the rehearsal includes a simulated sex scene, or nudity, to ensure the use of a closed set.

9. Onstage, when the performance includes a simulated sex scene, for an intimacy call to be held before each

performance. It is imperative the actors continue to rehearse, so they don't become careless and to ensure everyone feels secure and respected both onstage and off. The intimacy call is an opportunity to:

    a. Check in with the actors to ask how they think the intimacy and simulated sex scene went during the previous performance.

    b. Agreement and consent given for areas of physical touch before each performance, allowing for possible adaptations to be accommodated.

    c. Sculpting the physical actions using plain words, to be gone through at least twice.

10. On set, to employ a closed set as standard when filming simulated sex and nudity. Following the Closed Set Protocols, giving consideration to gender parity of the crew (i.e., female vulnerability in a heterosexual or lesbian intimate scene with an all-male crew).

11. Nudity. Any actor who has consented to nudity must make sure that their agent knows the actor wants a discussion about every nude scene and a summary of agreed scenes in writing. When working with nudity, for the Director to discuss the detail of every nude scene with the relevant actors, writing down the proposed shots and getting the actor's consent in writing. When working with nudity on set:

    a. Pre-agree times when nudity will be used.

    b. It is imperative to employ a closed set as standard when working with nudity.

    c. Nudity only from action to cut, and at all other times, the actor should be covered.

> d. No nudity with genitals touching. Always use patches or modesty barrier.

12. When kissing, no use of tongues as standard practice. However, should the Director feel it would serve the scene better to use tongues, then there must be agreement and consent from both of the actors. When rehearsing a stage/screen kiss,

> a. Start off with the actors giving and receiving a peck when agreeing physical touch, and sculpting the physical actions, using plain words,
>
> b. Then exploring the quality of the kiss when identifying the emotional content of the scene, and integrating the physical actions and emotional content.

13. Actors should not override the guidelines independently. Any new proposal is to be discussed with other actors and Director.

14. Consider the use of a suitably trained Intimacy Coordinator in scenes with simulated sexual content.

15. Scenes with simulated sex into abusive/violence simulated sexual content, consider the use of an Intimacy Coordinator in conjunction with a Fight Director/Stunt Coordinator.

With gratitude from Ita O'Brien, Founder, "Intimacy on Set": These guidelines would not have been possible without the work of Vanessa Ewan, Senior Lecturer and Course

Leader in Movement at the Royal Central School of Speech & Drama, in particular chapter 9 of her book *Actor Movement: Expression of the Physical Being* (Bloomsbury Methuen Drama, 2015), and her support in developing this approach. I am grateful to Meredith Dufton, previous Head of Movement at Mountview Academy of Theatre Arts, who invited me to teach the work to Mountview students in the Summer Term of 2015, which was instrumental in honing the guidelines. I would also like to thank Jennifer Ward-Lealand, President of New Zealand Equity, which was the first industry organization to adopt guidelines in this area; and Michael Hurst for sharing his working practice.

RESOURCES

ESSENTIAL READING

On Our Bodies

Bacon, L., *Health at Every Size: The Surprising Truth About Your Weight* (BenBella Books, 2010)

Hay, L. L., *You Can Heal Your Life* (Hay House, 1984)

Kapit, W., and Elson, L. M., *The Anatomy Coloring Book* (Pearson, 2013)

Mead, H., *Why Aren't We Talking About This?* (Square Peg, 2023)

Norman, L., and Cowan, T., *The Reflexology Handbook: A Complete Guide* (Piatkus, 2006)

Olsen, A., and McHose, C., *BodyStories: A Guide to Experiential Anatomy* (University Press of New England, 2004)

Pope, A., and Wurlitzer, S. H., *Wild Power: Discover the Magic of Your Menstrual Cycle and Awaken the Feminine Path to Power* (Hay House, 2017)

Tanner, R., *Step by Step Reflexology* (Douglas Barry Publications, 2003)

On Movement

Bainbridge-Cohen, B., *Sensing, Feeling, and Action: The Experiential Anatomy of Body-Mind Centering* (Contact Editions, 2003)

Conway, M., "Tea with Trish: The Movement Work of Trish Arnold" (DVD set)

Deniz and Guniz, "Eight Pieces of Brocades," Inarticulate Hour (August 31, 2019). Retrieved from: https://www.inarticulatehour .com/blog/2019/8/31/eight-pieces-of-brocades-also-known-as -ba-duan-jin-qi-gong-exercises

Ewan, V., and Green, D., *Actor Movement: Expression of the Physical Being* (Bloomsbury, 2014)

Farhi, D., *The Breathing Book: Good Health and Vitality Through Essential Breath Work* (Henry Holt, 1996)

Hartley, L., *Wisdom of the Body Moving: An Introduction to Body-Mind Centering* (North Atlantic Books, 1995)

Lecoq, J., *The Moving Body: Teaching Creative Theatre* (Metheuen Drama, 2009)

Marshall, L., *The Body Speaks: Performance and Expression* (Metheuen Drama, 2001)

Myers, T. W., *Anatomy Trains: Myofascial Meridians for Manual and Movement Therapies* (Elsevier, 2020)

Newlove, J., *Laban for Actors and Dancers* (Nick Hern Books, 2008)

Newlove, J., and Dalby, J., *Laban for All* (Nick Hern Books, 2003)

Roth, G., *Sweat Your Prayers: The Five Rhythms of the Soul* (Tarcher/ Putnam, 1998)

Suzuki, T., *The Way of Acting: The Theatre Writings of Tadashi Suzuki* (Theatre Communications Group, 1990)

On Fostering Intimacy

Ali, S., "Using Dance to Cultivate Self-Love." *Psychology Today*. 2022. https://www.psychologytoday.com/gb/blog/ a-modern-mentality/202202/using-dance-to-cultivate-self -love

Martin, B., and Dalzen, R., *The Art of Receiving and Giving: The Wheel of Consent* (Luminare Press, 2021)

McCormack, A., and McVeigh, S., "Behind the Famous '36 Questions That Lead to Love.'" Hack. ABC (March 26, 2017). Retrieved from: https://www.abc.net.au/triplej/programs/hack/ the-36-questions-that-lead-to-love/8387736

On Gender

Bates, L., *Everyday Sexism* (Simon & Schuster, 2014)

Cleghorn, E., *Unwell Women: A Journey Through Medicine and Myth in a Man-Made World* (W&N, 2021)

Gray, J., *Men Are from Mars, Women Are from Venus* (HarperCollins, 1992)

Jackson, G., *Pain and Prejudice* (Greystone Books Ltd, 2021)

Sangha, S. K., "The Invisibility of Women in Healthcare." Inspire the Mind. King's College London (March 8, 2024). Available at: https://www.inspirethemind.org/post/the-invisibility-of-women-in-healthcare

Sankey, E., " 'Deep in My Madness, Witches Gave Me Hope': Elizabeth Sankey on Motherhood, Depression and Witches." *Guardian* (November 24, 2024). Available at: https://www.theguardian.com/society/2024/nov/24/deep-in-my-madness-witches-gave-me-hope-elizabeth-sankey-on-motherhood-depression-and-witches

Sylvester, R., " 'The NHS Was Designed by Men for Men. My Role Is to Reset That.' " *The Times* (January 27, 2024). Available at: https://www.thetimes.com/uk/healthcare/article/the-nhs-was-designed-by-men-for-men-my-role-is-to-reset-that-82bhltxms

Thorpe, V., "What's Their Beef? Why Today's Leading Men Are Driven to Be Buff." *Guardian* (January 12, 2019). Retrieved from: https://www.theguardian.com/lifeandstyle/2019/jan/12/curse-of-perfection-male-actors-poldark

On Sex and Desire

"Anorgasmia in Women—Symptoms and Causes." Mayo Clinic (February 29, 2024). Available at: https://www.mayoclinic.org/diseases-conditions/anorgasmia/symptoms-causes/syc-20369422

Anonymous and Anderson, G., *Want* (Bloomsbury, 2024)

Comfort, A., and Quilliam, S., *The Joy of Sex: A Gourmet Guide to Lovemaking* (Mitchell Beazley, 2012)

Nagoski, E., *Come As You Are: The Surprising New Science That Will Transform Your Sex Life* (Scribe, 2015)

Neustädter, A., *Gayma Sutra: The Complete Guide to Sex Positions*
Newman, F., *The Whole Lesbian Sex Book: A Passionate Guide for All of Us* (Cleis Press, 2004)
Russell, S., and Kolb, J., *The Tao of Sexual Massage* (Gaia Books, 2000)
"Vaginismus: Causes, Symptoms, and Treatment." WebMD. Available at: https://www.webmd.com/women/vaginismus-causes-symptoms-treatments
Winston, S., *Women's Anatomy of Arousal: Secret Maps to Buried Pleasure* (Independently published, 2022)

On Parenting, Young People, and Sex Education
Blair, L., "No Sex Please; We're Parents" in Thompson, K., and McCann, D. (eds.) *Couples as Parents* (Routledge, 2024)
Keep It Real Online, "Keep It Real Online—Pornography," YouTube (June 6, 2020). Retrieved from: https://www.youtube.com/watch?v=94mINLDSWlk
Rivas-Lara, S., Kotecha, H., Pham, B., and Uhls, Y. T., "CSS Teens & Screens 2023: Romance or Nomance," Center for Scholars & Storytellers (2024)
Silverberg, C., and Smyth, F., *Sex Is a Funny Word: A Book About Bodies, Feelings and You* (Seven Stories Press, 2015)

Intimacy in Our Enchantress and Older Years
Ayres, S., and Eastman, M., "Sex, Intimacy and Sexual Wellbeing in Later Life," LLRC (15 Aug. 2022). Retrieved from: https://laterlifeaudioradio.org/news/sexuality-in-later-life-provocation-paper
Cox, T., *Great Sex Starts at 50: How to Age-Proof Your Libido*
Frostrup, M., and Smellie, A., *Cracking the Menopause: While Keeping Yourself Together* (Bluebird, 2021)
McCall, D., and Potter, N., *Menopausing: The Positive Roadmap to Your Second Spring* (HQ, 2002)
Pope, A., and Wurlitzer, S. H., *Wise Power* (Hay House, 2022)
"Senior Sex | What Can We Learn?" We-Vibe.com. 2025. https://www.we-vibe.com/uk/silversex
TED, "What Really Happens to Your Body During Menopause | Body Stuff with Dr. Jen Gunter," YouTube (June 10, 2021). Retrieved from: https://www.youtube.com/watch?v=cheqkrcHkrl

"The Age of Love." About. The Age of Love Consultancy. 2018.
 https://www.ageoflove.org/about
Wilkinson, A., "Jane Fonda, 86, Shares Exactly What Her Current
 Workout Routine Looks Like." *Women's Health*. December 20,
 2024. https://www.womenshealthmag.com/uk/fitness/
 a63245930/jane-fonda-workout-routine/

On Acting and Intimacy in the Media
Lets, E., "Why the Proper Representation of Female Pleasure on
 Television Matters," Her Campus (March 2, 2021). Retrieved
 from: https://www.hercampus.com/culture/female-pleasure
 -representation-television
Toomer, J., " 'Sex Education': How an Intimacy Coordinator Helped
 Change the Show's Approach to Love Scenes," *The Hollywood
 Reporter* (January 19, 2020) Retrieved from: https://www
 .hollywoodreporter.com/tv/tv-news/sex-education-howan
 -intimacy-coordinator-helped-change-shows-approach
 -lovescenes-1270697

On Spiritual Connection
Estés, C. P., *Women Who Run with the Wolves* (Rider, 2008)
Purce, J., *The Mystic Spiral* (Thames & Hudson, 2007)
Rutherford, L., *Principles of Shamanism* (Piatkus, 2014)
Strikes, T., and Orsi, J., *The Song of the Deer: The Great Sundance
 Journey of the Soul* (Jaguar Books, 1999)

FURTHER READING

Barker, M., *Rewriting the Rules: An Anti Self-Help Guide to Love,
 Sex and Relationships* (Routledge, 2012)
Bateman, V., *Naked Feminism: Breaking the Cult of Female Modesty*
 (Polity, 2023)
Bates, L., *Fix the System Not the Women* (Simon & Schuster,
 2022)
Benjamin, B. E., and Sohnen-Moe, C., *The Ethics of Touch* (Sohnen-
 Moe Associates, Inc., 2013)

Bettes, N., *Make Love Work: A Practical Guide to Relationship Success* (Allen & Unwin, 2024)

Blackie, S., *If Women Rose Rooted: The Power of the Celtic Woman* (September Publishing, 2016)

Bombadil, R., *Igniting Intimacy: Sex Magic Rituals for Radical Living and Loving.*

Boston, J., and Cook, R. (eds.), *Breath in Action: The Art of Breath in Vocal and Holistic Practice* (Jessica Kingsley Publishers, 2009)

Bown, A., *Dream Lovers: The Gamification of Relationships* (Pluto Press, 2022)

Boyle, K., *Everyday Pornography* (Routledge, 2010)

Boyle, K., *#MeToo, Weinstein and Feminism* (Palgrave, 2019)

Brochman, N., and Støkken Dahl, E., *The Wonder Down Under: The Ultimate Guide to Female Health and Empowerment* (Quercus, 2018)

Brotto, L. A., *Better Sex Through Mindfulness: How Women Can Cultivate Desire* (Greystone Books, 2018)

Brotto, L. A., *The Better Sex Through Mindfulness Workbook: A Guide to Cultivating Desire* (Greystone Books, 2022)

Brown, B., *Dare to Lead: Brave Work. Tough Conversations. Whole Hearts* (Penguin Random House, 2018)

Brunson, P. C., *Find Love: How to Navigate Modern Love and Discover the Right Partner for You* (Vermilion, 2024)

Bucher, J., *A Best Practice Guide to Sex and Storytelling: Filming Scenes with Sex and Nudity* (Routledge, 2018)

Carrellas, B., *Urban Tantra: Sacred Sex for the Twenty-First Century* (Ten Speed, 2017)

Chekhov, M., *To the Actor: On the Technique of Acting* (Routledge, 2002)

Crawford, P., *Blood, Bodies and Families in Early Modern England* (Routledge, 2004)

Dicks, J., *High Intensity Intercourse Training* (Pop Press, 2018)

Fake, S., *The Transgender Issue: An Argument for Justice* (Allen Lane, 2021)

Franklin, E., *Dynamic Alignment Through Imagery* (Human Kinetics Publishers, 1996)

Frantzis, B., *Opening the Energy Gates of Your Body: Qigong for Lifelong Health* (North Atlantic Books, 2005)

Gallagher, K., *The Goddess Path: 13 Steps to Becoming Your Most Intuitive, Authentic and Powerful Self* (Rider, 2024)

Hardy, J. W., and Easton, D., *The Ethical Slut* (Ten Speed, 2017)

hooks, b., *All About Love: New Visions* (HarperCollins, 2016)

Kaminoff, L., and Matthews, A., *Yoga Anatomy: Your Illustrated Guide to Postures, Movements and Breathing Techniques* (Human Kinetics, 2021)

Kleinplatz, L. P., and Menard, A. D., *Magnificent Sex: Lessons from Extraordinary Lovers* (Routledge, 2020)

Koch, L., *The Psoas Book* (Guinea Pig Publications, 1997)

Laffy, G., *Love Sex: An Integrative Model for Sexual Education* (Routledge, 2023)

Lee, N., *Feeling Myself: How I Shed My Shame to Find Sexual Freedom and You Can Too* (Vermilion, 2022)

Leight, A., and Mercree, C., *A Little Bit of Chakras: An Introduction to Energy Healing* (Sterling Ethos, 2016)

Leyden, K. M., et al., "Walkable Neighborhoods," *Journal of the American Planning Association* (April 11, 2023), 90 (1): 1–14.

Lister, K., *A Curious History of Sex* (Unbound, 2020)

Malone, A., *The Female Gaze: Essential Movies Made by Women* (TMA Press, 2018)

Marqarot, H., *Reflex Zone Therapy on the Feet: A Textbook for Therapists* (Churchill Livingstone, 2000)

Moyle, K., *The Science of Sex: Every Question About Your Sex Life Answered* (DK, 2023)

Oliver, K., *Hunting Girls: Sexual Violence from* The Hunger Games *to Campus Rape* (Columbia University Press, 2016)

Olsen, A., *Body and Earth: An Experiential Guide* (Wesleyan University Press, 2020)

Olsen, A., *Moving Between Worlds: A Guide to Embodied Living and Community* (Wesleyan University Press, 2022)

Olsen, A., *The Place of Dance* (Wesleyan University Press, 2014)

Perez, C. C., *Invisible Women: Exposing Data and Bias in a World Designed for Men* (Chatto & Windus, 2019)

Pine, E., *Notes to Self* (Penguin, 2019)

Price, J., *Naked at Our Age: Talking Out Loud About Senior Sex* (Seal Press, 2011)

Redmond, L., *When the Drummers Were Women: A Spiritual History of Rhythm* (Echo Point Books & Media, 2018)

Reyneke, D., *Ultimate Pilates: Achieve the Perfect Body Shape* (Vermilion, 2002)

Richardson, D., *Tantric Orgasm for Women* (Destiny Books, 2004)

Richardson, D., *The Heart of Tantric Sex: A Unique Guide to Love and Sexual Fulfillment* (O-Books, 2003)

Roth, G., *Maps to Ecstasy: A Healing Journey for the Untamed Spirit* (Thorsons, 1999)

Rotman, I., and Corinna, H., *Wait, What?: A Comic Guide to Relationships, Bodies and Growing Up* (Oni Press, 2019)

Saradananda, S., *The Power of Breath: The Art of Breathing Well for Harmony, Happiness and Health* (Watkins Publishing, 2009)

Scaravelli, V., *Awakening the Spine* (Pinter & Martin, 2011)

Sile, B., *The Pilates Body: The Ultimate At-Home Guide to Strengthening, Lengthening and Toning Your Body Without Machines* (Harmony, 2000)

Simon, R. E., and Grigni, N., *The Every Body Book: The LGBTQ+ Inclusive Guide for Kids About Sex, Gender, Bodies, and Families* (Jessica Kingsley Publishers, 2020)

Smith Galer, S., *Losing It: Dispelling the Sex Myths That Rule Our Lives* (William Collins, 2022)

Soma, S., *Everyone's Invited* (Gallery UK, 2022)

Srinivasan, A., *The Right to Sex* (Bloomsbury, 2021)

Starck, M., *Women's Medicine Ways: Cross-Cultural Rites of Passage* (Crossing Press, 1993)

Staugaard-Jones, J. A., *The Vital Psoas Muscle: Connecting Physical, Emotional and Spiritual Well-Being* (Lotus Publishing Ltd., 2012)

Stone, L., *The Family, Sex and Marriage in England 1500–1800* (Penguin, 1990)

Thorburn, M., and Powling, S., *The Relate Guide to Loving in Later Life: Intimacy in the Prime of Life* (Vermilion, 2000)

Trafford, L. J., *Sex and Sexuality in Ancient Rome* (Pen & Sword History, 2021)

Tsiara, A., and Werth, B., *The Architecture and Design of Man and Woman* (Doubleday, 2004)

Tufnell, M., and Crickmay, C., *Body Space Image: Notes Toward Improvisation and Performance* (Triarchy Press, 2023)

Van der Kolk, B., *The Body Keeps the Score: Mind, Brain and Body in the Transformation of Trauma* (Penguin, 2015)

Williams, L. R., *The Erotic Thriller in Contemporary Cinema* (Edinburgh University Press, 2005)

Williamson, M., *A Return to Love: Reflections on the Principles of a Course in Miracles* (HarperCollins, 1996)

NOTES

Prologue: An Intimate Scene

1 Ramachandran, N., " 'Normal People' Creators, Actors Reveal Intimacy Process," *Variety* (August 26, 2020). Retrieved from: https://variety.com/2020/tv/global/normal-people-intimacy-daisy-edgar-jones-paul-mescal-1234749207/

2 Handler, R., "How *Normal People* Does Sex So Good," *Vulture* (April 30, 2020). Retrieved from: https://www.vulture.com/2020/04/normal-people-good-sex-scenes.html

Chapter One: The Mirror

1 *Brainwashed: Sex-Camera-Power*, documentary directed by Nina Menkes (2022)

2 Wiegand, C., "Top Stars Must Help Protect Cast and Crew from Bad Behavior, Says Denise Gough," *Guardian* (March 11, 2024). Retrieved from: https://www.theguardian.com/stage/2024/mar/11/denise-gough-people-places-and-things

3 Lawson, M., "Gemma Whelan: 'Sex in *Game of Thrones* Could Be a Frenzied Mess,' " *Guardian* (November 2, 2024). Retrieved from: https://www.theguardian.com/tv-and-radio/2021/nov/02/gemma-whelan-sex-game-of-thrones-frenzied-mess-tower-innuendo

4 Brown, M., "Baftas 2021: Michaela Coel Dedicates Win to Intimacy Coordinator," *Guardian* (June 6, 2021). Retrieved from:

https://www.theguardian.com/culture/2021/jun/06/baftas-2021
-michaela-coel-dedicates-win-to-intimacy-coordinator
5 The Everyday Sexism Project. Available at: https://
everydaysexism.com/
6 Bates, L., *Everyday Sexism* (Simon & Schuster, 2019)
7 Ewan, V., and Green, D., "Personal Safety in Movement" in *Actor Movement: Expression of the Physical Being* (Bloomsbury, 2014)

Chapter Two: What Do I Want?
1 "What Gen Z Don't Get About Love," *The Times* (September 27, 2022). Retrieved from: https://www.thetimes.co.uk/article/hinge
-justin-mcleod-gen-z-love-dating-romance-xbpwdfgzj
2 Teen Dating Violence Month, https://www.teendvmonth.org/
3 Weaver, M., "Mark Rylance Pulls Out of Three Jerusalem Shows After Brother's Death," *Guardian* (June 10, 2022). Retrieved from: https://www.theguardian.com/culture/2022/jun/10/mark
-rylance-pulls-out-of-three-jerusalem-shows-after-brothers-death
4 "How the Covid-19 Lockdowns Affected the Domestic Abuse Crisis," UK Research and Innovation (August 12, 2022). Retrieved from: https://www.ukri.org/who-we-are/how-we-are
-doing/research-outcomes-and-impact/esrc/how-the-covid-19
-lockdowns-affected-the-domestic-abuse-crisis/
5 Retrieved from: BBC Newsbeat, "Porn: The 'Incredible' Number of UK Adults Watching Content," BBC (June 11, 2021). Retrieved from: https://www.bbc.co.uk/news/newsbeat
-57428077; Robb-Dover, K., "Revealing Statistics Re: Pornography Addiction," FHEHealth (July 21, 2024). Retrieved from: https://fherehab.com/learning/pornography-addiction
-stats
6 Saner, E., "The Rise of Voluntary Celibacy: 'Most of the Sex I've Had, I Wish I Hadn't Bothered'," *Guardian* (April 26, 2023). Retrieved from: https://www.theguardian.com/lifeandstyle/
2023/apr/26/the-rise-of-voluntary-celibacy-most-of-the-sex-ive
-had-i-wish-i-hadnt-bothered
7 Ibid.

Chapter Three: The First Steps Toward Intimacy

1 Krznaric, R., "The Ancient Greeks' 6 Words for Love (And Why Knowing Them Can Change Your Life)," *Yes!* (December 28, 2023). Retrieved from: https://www.yesmagazine.org/health -happiness/2013/12/28/the-ancient-greeks-6-words-for-love-and -why-knowing-them-can-change-your-life

2 Smiljkovic, I., "Marina & Ulay @ MoMA (The Artist Is Present)," YouTube (November 2, 2012). Retrieved from: https://www .youtube.com/watch?v=xlf68X2qEpM

3 Pegg, M., "J is for Sidney Jourard: His Work on the Transparent Self," *The Positive Encourager* (August 6, 2024). Retrieved from: https://www.thepositiveencourager.global/sidney-jourards -approach-to-doing-positive-work/

4 Prigg, M., "The iPad Really IS Child's Play: More Than Half of Toddlers Can Use Apple's Tablet When They Are Just ONE, Researchers Say," *Daily Mail* (July 4, 2015). Retrieved from: https://www.dailymail.co.uk/sciencetech/article-3149025/

5 Eunice Kennedy Shriver National Institute of Child Health and Human Development (NICHD), "High Amounts of Screen Time Begin as Early as Infancy, NIH Study Suggests," *National Institutes of Health* (November 25, 2019). Retrieved from: https://www.nih.gov/news-events/news-releases/high-amounts -screen-time-begin-early-infancy-nih-study-suggests

6 Guthold, R., et al., "Global Trends in Insufficient Physical Activity Among Adolescents: A Pooled Analysis of 298 Population-Based Surveys with 1.6 Million Participants," *Lancet Child & Adolescent Health* (2020), doi: 10:1016/S2352-4642(19)30323-2

7 Chevalier, G., et al., "Earthing: Health Implications of Reconnecting the Human Body to the Earth's Surface Electrons," *Journal of Environmental and Public Health* (2012), doi: 10:1155/2012/291541

8 Bainbridge Cohen, B., *Sensing, Feeling, and Action: The Experiential Anatomy of Body-Mind Centering* (Wesleyan University Press, 2021)

9 Hartley, L., *Wisdom of the Body Moving: An Introduction to Body-Mind Centering* (North Atlantic Books, 1995), p. 215

10 Bhardwaj, C., "Want Real, True Sexual Energy? Look to Your Root Chakra," Chandresh Bhardwaj (July 14, 2017). Retrieved from: https://cbmeditates.com/blog-post/2015/7/14/want-real -true-sexual-energy-look-to-your-root-chakra

11 *Wisdom of the Body Moving*, p. 214

12 *Wisdom of the Body Moving*, p. 219

13 Bureau, Zee Media, "Stress Reduction to Improved Sleep: 7 Benefits of Walking Barefoot on Grass," Zee News (November 5, 2023). https://zeenews.india.com/health/ stressreduction-toimproved-sleep-7-benefits-of-walking -barefootongrass-2684415; and "What Is Grounding and Can It Help Improve Your Health?", Healthline (August 30, 2019).

14 Bureau, Zee Media, "Stress reduction to improved sleep."

Chapter Four: Seeing Ourselves

1 Ravindran, M., "Emma Thompson Charms Berlin with 'Leo Grande,' Speaks Candidly About Women Being 'Brainwashed' to Hate Their Bodies," *Variety* (February 12, 2022). Retrieved from: https://variety.com/2022/film/global/emma-thompson -women-bodies-brainwashed-1235180029/

2 Gao, M., "Emma Thompson's New Movie Puts Aging and Sexuality into a Revolutionary New Light," *Harper's Bazaar* (June 22, 2022). Retrieved from: https://www.harpersbazaar .com/culture/film-tv/a40379241/emma-thompson-daryl -mccormack-good-luck-leo-grande-interview/

3 Light, A., "It's Okay to Feel Hurt When Celebrities Lose Weight—but Let's Unpack It," *Glamour* (February 24, 2025). Retrieved from: https://www.glamourmagazine.co.uk/article/ celebrity-weight-loss

4 Mahanty, S., "ELLE Style Awards: Florence Pugh Is the British Icon," *ELLE* (August 30, 2023). Retrieved from: https://www.elle .com/uk/life-and-culture/culture/a44863369/florence-pugh -interview-elle-style-awards/

5 Durney, S., "Florence Pugh Addressed a 'Weird' Rumor About Her Transformation for 'We Live in Time,'" BuzzFeed

(September 6, 2024). Retrieved from: https://www.buzzfeed
.com/ellendurney/florence-pugh-on-shaved-head-for-we-live-in
-time

6 Etcoff, N., et al., "The Real Truth About Beauty: A Global
Report," *Club of Amsterdam* (2004). https://www
.clubofamsterdam.com/contentarticles/52%20Beauty/dove
_white_paper_final.pdf

7 Children's Commissioner, "Young People with Eating Disorders
in England on the Rise," Children's Commissioner (August 1,
2023). Retrieved from: https://www.childrenscommissioner.gov
.uk/blog/young-people-with-eating-disorders-in-england-on-the
-rise/

8 Venti, L., "Here's Why I Wore Makeup to Bed for Almost 1 Year,"
Cosmopolitan (March 3, 2016). Retrieved from: https://www
.cosmopolitan.com/style-beauty/beauty/a54664/i-wore-makeup
-to-bed-for-my-boyfriend/

9 Sawyer, M., " 'I Stripped Away This Caricature That I Created':
Pamela Anderson on Makeup, Activism and Gardening,"
Guardian (February 23, 2025). Retrieved from: https://www
.theguardian.com/culture/2025/feb/23/pamela-anderson
-baywatch-last-showgirl-liam-neeson

10 Meale, C., "Chloë Grace Moretz on Fame and Social Media:
'I Basically Became a Recluse,' " *Hunger* (September 20, 2022).
Retrieved from: https://hungermag.com/editorial/chloe-grace
-moretz-on-fame-and-social-media-i-basically-became-a-recluse

11 Milmo, D., and Hern, A., "TikTok Self-Harm Study Results 'Every
Parent's Nightmare,' " *Guardian* (December 15, 2022). Retrieved
from: https://www.theguardian.com/technology/2022/dec/15/
tiktok-self-harm-study-results-every-parents-nightmare

12 White, A., "Channing Tatum on the Female Perspective in
'Magic Mike 3' and Why Training for His Role Is 'Unhealthy,' "
The Hollywood Reporter (February 19, 2022). Retrieved from:
https://www.hollywoodreporter.com/movies/movie-news/
channing-tatum-magic-mike-3-female-perspective-unhealthy
-training-1235096752/

13 Mazziotta, J., "Robert Pattinson Was 'Counting Sips of Water'

Before Shooting Shirtless Scenes for 'The Batman,' " *People* (March 2, 2022). Retrieved from: https://people.com/health/robert-pattinson-was-counting-sips-of-water-before-shirtless-scenes-for-the-batman/

14 Horowitz, J., "Kate Winslet Talks AVATAR: THE WAY OF WATER, TITANIC, & More!," YouTube (December 16, 2022). Retrieved from: https://www.youtube.com/watch?v=L22JpW6an-o

15 Hello!, "Retouching Is 'Excessive' Says Slimline Covergirl Kate Winslet," *Hello!* (January 9, 2003). Retrieved from: https://www.hellomagazine.com/film/20030110510987/katewinslet/

16 Dowd, Maureen, "Kate Winslet Has No Filter," *New York Times* (May 31, 2021). Retrieved from: https://www.nytimes.com/2021/05/31/style/mare-of-easttown-kate-winslet.html

17 Nugent, A., "Anne-Marie Duff Speaks Out About Decision Not to Get Botox: 'Some People Think It's Bonkers,' " *Independent* (May 22, 2022). Retrived from: https://www.independent.co.uk/arts-entertainment/theatre-dance/news/anne-marie-duff-botox-b2082952.html

18 NPR Staff, "Like Olive Kitteridge, Actress Frances McDormand Was Tired of Supporting Roles," NPR (October 31, 2014). Retrieved from: https://www.npr.org/2014/10/31/360183633/like-olive-kitteridge-actress-frances-mcdormand-was-tired-of-supporting-roles

19 Dean, J., "Kate Winslet: 'My Daughter's Generation Can Speak for Themselves,' " *The Times* (December 3, 2022). Retrieved from: https://www.thetimes.com/culture/article/kate-winslet-daughter-i-am-ruth-interview-f2663bpt7

20 HeartMath Institute, "Energetic Communication," *Science of the Heart: Exploring the Role of the Heart in Human Performance* (2016). Retrieved from: https://www.heartmath.org/research/science-of-the-heart/energetic-communication/

21 Katz-Wise, S. L., "Gender Fluidity: What It Means and Why Support Matters," Harvard Health Publishing (December 3, 2020). Retrieved from: https://www.health.harvard.edu/blog/gender-fluidity-what-it-means-and-why-support-matters 2020120321544

22 Mace, L., "Wonder Down Under: The Vagina Myths Exposed - Ellen Stokken Dahl & Nina Brochmann (live interview)," YouTube (May 31, 2018). Retrieved from: https://www.youtube .com/watch?v=Fp4Zbj26PPc

23 Women's Health Victoria, "New Research Finds Porn and Online Media Are Fuelling Significant Anxiety Around Genital Appearance Among Young Women in Australia," Women's Health Victoria (June 17, 2024). Retrieved from: https://whv.org .au/resources/whv-publications/new-research-finds-porn-and -online-media-are-fuelling-significant-anxiety

24 Harvey-Jenner, C., and Williams, S., " 'Is My Vagina Normal?' Yes! Here Are the 7 Different Types of Vaginas," *Cosmopolitan* (October 21, 2024). Retrieved from: https://www.cosmopolitan .com/uk/body/health/g11658368/is-my-vagina-normal-shape -size-vulva-labia/

25 Hibberd, J., " 'Naked Attraction' Boss responds to U.S. Controversy, Explains Nude Casting Process," *The Hollywood Reporter* (October 2, 2023). Retrieved from: https://www .hollywoodreporter.com/tv/tv-news/naked-attraction-boss -casting-controversy-interview-1235604435/

26 Harvey, L., "Why I Photographed 100 Vulvas," BBC (February 11, 2019). Retrieved from: https://www.bbc.co.uk/ news/resources/idt-sh/Why_I_Photographed_100_Vulvas

27 Nagoski, E., *Come as You Are* (Scribe, 2015)

Chapter Five: Calling Our Boundaries, Giving Consent

 1 Babalola, B., "The Innate Black Britishness of *'I May Destroy You,'* " *Vulture* (August 3, 2020). Retrieved from: https://www .vulture.com/article/i-may-destroy-you-black-britishness.html

 2 Davies, H. J., "I May Destroy You: Why Michaela Coel's Drama Is a True TV Gamechanger," *Guardian* (July 11, 2020). Retrieved from: https://www.theguardian.com/tv-and-radio/2020/jul/11/i -may-destroy-you-why-michaela-coels-drama-is-a-true-tv -gamechanger

 3 #consentiseverything, https://www.consentiseverything.com/

 4 Gloucestershire Healthy Living and Learning, "Keep Breathing,"

YouTube (March 23, 2022). Retrieved from: https://www.youtube
.com/watch?v=TnSEkiiUlmA

5 1in6, https://1in6.org/statistic/

6 Kolmar, C., "17 Distressing Sexual Harassment Statistics: Sexual
   Harassment in the Workplace," Zippia (July 10, 2023). Retrieved
   from: https://www.zippia.com/advice/sexual-harassment
   -workplace-statistics

7 "LGBT People Nearly Four Times More Likely Than Non LGBT
   People to Be Victims of Violent Crime," UCLA School of Law,
   Williams Institute (October 2, 2020). Retrieved from: https://
   williamsinstitute.law.ucla.edu/press/ncvs-lgbt-violence-press
   -release/

8 "Sexual Harassment in Our Nation's Workplaces," U.S. Equal
   Employment Opportunity Commission (April 2022). Retrieved
   from: https://www.eeoc.gov/data/sexual-harassment-our-nations
   -workplaces; "The Facts Behind the #MeToo Movement: A
   National Study on Sexual Harassment and Assault," Stop Street
   Harassment (2018). Retrieved from: https://www.stopstreet
   harassment.org/wp-content/uploads/2018/01/Survey
   -Questions-2018-National-Study-on-Sexual-Harassment-and
   -Assault.pdf

9 "Domestic Abuse Victim Characteristics, England and Wales:
   Year Ending March 2023," Office for National Statistics
   (November 24, 2023). Retrieved from: https://www.ons.gov.uk/
   peoplepopulationandcommunity/crimeandjustice/articles/
   domesticabusevictimcharacteristicsenglandandwales/
   yearendingmarch2023

10 Martin, B., "The Wheel of Consent," BettyMartin.org. Retrieved
   from: https://bettymartin.org/

11 Pickard, M., "Intimate Relations," *Drama Quarterly* (April 28, 2020).
   Retrieved from: https://dramaquarterly.com/intimate-relations/

12 "Alfred Tomatis Research and Legacy," Tomatis. Retrieved from:
   https://www.tomatis.com/en/alfred-tomatis

13 Catalfo, P., "Beyond Words," *New Age Journal* (November/
   December 1986). Retrieved from: https://www.jillpurce.com/
   articles-by-or-about-jill-purce/beyond-words

14 Sue Appleby, https://www.sueappleby.co.uk/

15 Betty Martin, https://bettymartin.org/

Chapter Six: The Sensuous Body

1 Sundance Institute, "Power of Story: On Intimacy," YouTube (February 8, 2023). Retrieved from: https://www.youtube.com/watch?v=j7_35oEldNk

2 Dean, J., "Florence Pugh: 'I've Watched Talented, Beautiful Women Get Torn Apart,'" *The Times* (December 15, 2024). Retrieved from: https://www.thetimes.com/culture/film/article/florence-pugh-interview-we-live-in-time-p8pr8zpls

3 Enrico Cuini, https://www.enricocuini.com/about

4 O'Brien, I., and Green, D., "From Grounded Foot to Leaping Foot" (June 19, 2011)

5 Suzuki, T., and Rimer, J. T., *The Way of Acting* (Theatre Communications Group Inc., 1990), p. 8

6 Persis Jadé Maravala, https://beyondconference.org/archive/b23/speakers/persis-jade-maravala.html

Chapter Seven: Connection and Communication

1 Harris, J., "In an Isolated World, Humans Need to Dance Together More Than Ever—but We're Running Out of Places to Do It," *Guardian* (March 19, 2020). Retrieved from: https://www.theguardian.com/commentisfree/2023/mar/19/isolated-humans-dance-together-demise-clubbing; Davies, R., "'It's Not Just a Dancefloor': The Precipitous Decline of UK Nightclubs," *Guardian* (December 27, 2024). Retrieved from: https://www.theguardian.com/business/2024/dec/27/calls-to-save-the-uks-ailing-nightclub-industry-after-another-year-of-closures

2 Gabrielle Roth's 5Rhythms, https://www.5rhythms.com/gabrielle-roths-5rhythms/

3 Leo Rutherford, https://eagleswing.co.uk/about-eagles-wing/eagles-wing-practioners/leo-rutherford-biography/

4 5Rhythms, https://www.5rhythms.com/gabrielle-roths-5rhythms/

5 "Covid Lockdown." News in Reproduction. Focus on Reproduction. https://www.focusonreproduction.eu/article/News-in-Reproduction-COVID-lockdown

6 Newman, F., *The Whole Lesbian Sex Book: A Passionate Guide For All of Us* (Cleis Press, 1999)

7 Neustädter, A., *Gayma Sutra: The Complete Guide to Sex Positions* (Bruno Gmünder, 2014)

8 Kaur, T., "Queer Representation in Media: The Good, the Bad, and the Ugly," Heckin' Unicorn Blog (October 14, 2023). Retrieved from: https://heckinunicorn.com/blogs/heckin-unicorn-blog/queer -representation-in-media-comprehensive-list-breakdown-lgbt

9 Snow, J., "Trish Arnold Obituary," *Guardian* (February 27, 2017). Retrieved from: https://www.theguardian.com/lifeandstyle/ 2017/feb/27/trish-arnold-obituary

Chapter Eight: The Myth and Reality of Sexual Arousal

1 Moran, C., "Emma Thompson: Why I'm Going Naked at 63," *The Times* (May 20, 2022). Retrieved from: https://www .thetimes.co.uk/article/emma-thompson-why-im-going-naked-at -63-bmlw7rgpc

2 Schager, N., "Marvel Is Weird About Sex," *Esquire* (November 11, 2021). Retrieved from: https://www.esquire.com/ entertainment/a38222234/marvel-eternals-weird-about-sex/

3 Benedict, R. S., "Everyone Is Beautiful and No One Is Horny," *Blood Knife* (February 14, 2021). Retrieved from: https:// bloodknife.com/everyone-beautiful-noone-horny/

4 Conn, A., and Hodges, K. R., "Genito-Pelvic Pain/Penetration Disorder" in *MSD Manual Professional Version* (2023). Retrieved from: https://www.msdmanuals.com/professional/gynecology -and-obstetrics/female-sexual-function-and-dysfunction/genito -pelvic-pain-penetration-disorder

5 Cook, S., "I Watched BBC's Men Up and It's a Heartwarming Rollercoaster That's a Real Life Lesson to Us Men," Wales Online (December 29, 2023). Retrieved from: https://www .walesonline.co.uk/lifestyle/tv/watched-bbcs-men-up-its -28360128

6 Smith, E. W., "What *Sex Education* Gets Right About Vaginismus," *Refinery29* (January 22, 2020). Retrieved from: https://www.refinery29.com/en-gb/2020/01/9256514/what-is -vaginismus-sex-education-lily-season-2-episode-8

7 "Overview: Premature Ejaculation," Institute for Quality and Efficiency in Health Care (IQWiG) (2006). Retrieved from: https://www.ncbi.nlm.nih.gov/books/NBK547548/

8 Sharman, L. S., Fitzgerald, R., and Douglas, H., "Prevalence of Sexual Strangulation/Choking Among Australian 18–35 Year-Olds," *Archives of Sexual Behavior* (2024). doi.org/10:1007/s10508-024-02937-y

9 Kissane, K., "Study Finds Strangling During Sex Common, but Understanding Is Low," University of Melbourne (July 2, 2024). Retrieved from: https://www.unimelb.edu.au/newsroom/news/2024/july/study-finds-strangling-during-sex-common,-but-understanding-is-low

10 Thomas, M., *The Good Sex Project* [podcast]

11 Moorhead, J., "Never Go to Bed on an Argument . . . and 19 Other Relationship 'Rules' Unpicked by Experts," *Guardian* (June 9, 2023). Retrieved from: https://www.theguardian.com/lifeandstyle/2023/jun/09/therapists-reveal-20-truths-and-myths-about-relationships

12 Bale, M., "Donald Sutherland on His Famous *Don't Look Now* Sex Scene," *Vulture* (March 6, 2018). Retrieved from: https://www.vulture.com/2018/03/donald-sutherland-on-his-famous-dont-look-now-sex-scene.htm

13 Richmond, T., "Behind the Scenes on Don't Look Now: A Photo Retrospective of the Cinematic Great," *Empire* (June 29, 2011). Retrieved from: https://www.empireonline.com/movies/features/behind-scenes-dont-look-now/

Chapter Nine: Sex Education

1 De Souza, R., "'A Lot of It Is Actually Just Abuse'—Young People and Pornography," Children's Commissioner (January 31, 2023). Retrieved from: https://www.childrenscommissioner.gov.uk/resource/a-lot-of-it-is-actually-just-abuse-young-people-and-pornography/

2 Jhe, G. B., Addison, J., Lin, J., and Pluhar, E., "Pornography Use Among Adolescents and the Role of Primary Care." *Family Medicine and Community Health* 11 (1): e001776. https://fmch.bmj.com/content/11/1/e001776

3 Active* Consent, https://www.consenthub.ie/

4 Ide, W., "How to Have Sex Review—Two Stars Are Born with This Searing Study of Consent," *Guardian* (November 5, 2023). Retrieved from: https://www.theguardian.com/film/2023/nov/05/how-to-have-sex-review-two-stars-are-born-in-a-searing-study-of-consent-molly-manning-walker-mia-mckenna-bruce

5 McLean, C., "Mia McKenna-Bruce Interview: How to Have Sex Star on Consent and Porn," *The Standard* (November 4, 2023). Retrieved from. https://www.standard.co.uk/culture/film/mia-mckenna-bruce-interview-how-to-have-sex-consent-b1118079.html

6 School Consent Project, https://www.schoolsconsentproject.com/

7 Hislop, M., "Consent Education to Become Mandatory in All Schools from 2023." Women's Agenda (February 17, 2022). https://womensagenda.com.au/latest/consent-education-to-become-mandatory-in-all-schools-from-2023/

8 Thorpe, N., Barbu, M., and Kirby, P., "Tate Brothers Arrive in US After Romania Prosecutors Lift Travel Ban," *BBC News* (February 27, 2025). Retrieved from: https://www.bbc.co.uk/news/articles/cpq222rqv4po

9 Oppenheim, M., "TikTok 'Failing to Act' as Andrew Tate Videos Still Seen by Children as Young as 13," *Independent* (July 2, 2023). Retrieved from: https://www.independent.co.uk/news/uk/home-news/andrew-tate-tristan-videos-tiktok-b2362496.html

10 "Who Is Andrew Tate?" Center for Countering Digital Hate (June 30, 2023). Retrieved from: https://counterhate.com/blog/who-is-andrew-tate-influencer-misogyny-women-hate/

11 *Sensing, Feeling and Action*, p. 39

12 "I: Spider-Man Star Andrew Garfield on Why He's Standing Up for Male Sexual Abuse Victims in 'Therapeutic' Play." Intimacy on Set (2023). https://www.intimacyonset.com/press/i-spider-man-star-andrew-garfield-on-why-hes-standing-up-for-male-sexual-abuse-victims-in-therapeutic-play

Chapter Ten: A Lifetime of Intimate Relationships

1 Green, E., "Consent Isn't Enough: The Troubling Sex of *Fifty Shades*," *The Atlantic* (February 10, 2015). Retrieved from: https://www.theatlantic.com/culture/archive/2015/02/consent -isnt-enough-in-fifty-shades-of-grey/385267/

2 maude, https://getmaude.com/pages/ethos

3 Regensdorf, L., "Dakota Johnson and Maude Are Ready to Make Sex More Beautiful," *Vanity Fair* (2020). Retrieved from: https://www.vanityfair.com/style/2020/11/dakota-johnson-joins -maude-sexual-wellness

4 Len Catron, M., "To Fall in Love with Anyone, Do This," *New York Times* (January 9, 2015). Retrieved from: https://www .nytimes.com/2015/01/11/style/modern-love-to-fall-in-love-with -anyone-do-this.html

5 Miranda Harcourt discusses this in a January 2021 edition of her subscriber-only Substack account, "Notes on Actors," https:// mirandaharcourt.substack.com/p/notes-for-actors-2f0

6 Red School, https://www.redschool.net/wildpower

7 Figes, K., and Zimmerman, J., *Life After Birth: What Even Your Friends Won't Tell You About Motherhood* (Golden Books, 2001)

8 "Changes in Your Relationships After Having a Baby," NCT (2022). Retrieved from: https://www.nct.org.uk/life-parent/your -relationship-couple/relationship-changes/changes-your -relationships-after-having-baby

9 Ryan R. A., "Intimacy," Movers and Shakers (2025). Retrieved from: https://www.moversandshakerspodcast.com/post/ intimacy

10 Cain Carroll, C., and Kimata, L., *Partner Yoga: Making Contact for Physical, Emotional, and Spiritual Growth* (Rodale Press, 2000)

Chapter Eleven: Finding the Enchantress

1 Rogers, J., "Greta Scacchi: 'I Was Always Being Invited to Play a Male Fantasy,'" *Guardian* (November 12, 2023). Retrieved from: https://www.theguardian.com/film/2023/nov/12/greta-scacchi -she-stoops-to-conquer-orange-tree-richmond-interview

2 Wojciechowski, M., "Andie MacDowell: Loving Her Age," Next Avenue (December 6, 2022). Retrieved from: https://www .nextavenue.org/andie-macdowell-influencer-in-aging/

3 "Menopause in the Workplace," NHS England (March 9, 2022). Retrieved from: https://www.engage.england.nhs.uk/safety-and -innovation/menopause-in-the-workplace/#:~:text=It%20is %20estimated%20that%20there,can%20last%20for%20several %20years

4 "BMS & WHC's 2020 Recommendations on Hormone Replacement Therapy in Menopausal Women," British Menopause Society (2023). Retrieved from: https://thebms.org .uk/wp-content/uploads/2023/10/02-BMS-ConsensusStatement -BMS-WHC-2020-Recommendations-on-HRT-in-menopausal -women-SEPT2023-A.pdf

5 "BMS Comment on Channel 4 Program: Davina McCall: Sex, Myths and the Menopause," British Menopause Society (May 3, 2022). Retrieved from: https://thebms.org.uk/2022/05/bms -comment-on-channel-4-program-davina-mccall-sex-myths-and -the-menopause/

6 "Importance of Managing Menopause," Clinical Reviews (2025). Retrieved from: https://clinical-reviews.com/uk/supplements/ menopause

7 Wilkinson, A., "Jane Fonda, 86, Shares Exactly What Her Current Workout Routine Looks Like," Women's Health (December 20, 2024). Retrieved from: https://www .womenshealthmag.com/uk/fitness/a63245930/jane-fonda -workout-routine/

8 "The 'Male Menopause,'" NHS (October 13, 2022). Retrieved from: https://www.nhs.uk/conditions/male-menopause/

9 BBC Three. "Why You Should Look Forward to the Menopause | Fleabag Series 2," YouTube (2019). Retrieved from: https://www .youtube.com/watch?v=RZrnHnASRV8

10 Steckenrider, J., "Sexual Activity of Older Adults: Let's Talk About It," The Lancet 4(3) (2023). Retrieved from: https://www .thelancet.com/journals/lanhl/article/PIIS2666-7568(23)00003-X/ fulltext#back-bib4

11 Kelly, Sarah-Louise, "Pleasure Has No Age Limit—We're Still Having Sex in Our 80s." HuffPost UK (August 11, 2023). https://www.huffingtonpost.co.uk/entry/pleasure-has-no-age-limit-were-still-having-sex-in-our-80s_uk_64d5e90de4b03368db1e2af4

12 Ayres, S., and Eastman, M. (eds.), "Sex, Intimacy and Sexual Wellbeing in Later Life." The Age Action Alliance (2022). Available at: https://theageactionalliance.org/wp-content/uploads/2022/12/Sex-Intimacy-pages-11082022-FINAL.pdf

13 Ibid.

14 Shoichet, C. E., and Leipzig, P., "More Baby Boomers Are Living Alone. One Reason Why: 'Gray Divorce,'" CNN (August 5, 2023). Retrieved from: https://edition.cnn.com/2023/08/05/health/boomers-divorce-living-alone-wellness-cec/index.html

15 Willen, C., "'The Great' Intimacy Coordinator Wants More Kissing for Old Characters." Business Insider (December 9, 2021). Retrieved from: https://www.businessinsider.com/the-great-intimacy-coordinator-older-characters-sex-kissing-katharine-hardman-2021-12

16 Murray, N., "'The Last of Us' Season 1, Episode 3 Recap: One More Good Day," New York Times (January 29, 2023). Retrieved from: https://www.nytimes.com/2023/01/29/arts/television/the-last-of-us-recap-episode-3.html

17 Watson, I., "Ad of the Day: Rankin and Relate's Ode to Joy of Later Life Sex," The Drum (April 26, 2021). Retrieved from: https://www.thedrum.com/news/2021/04/26/ad-the-day-rankin-and-relate-s-ode-joy-later-life-sex

18 "Let's Talk the Joy of Sex in Later Life," Relate. Retrieved from: https://www.relate.org.uk/lets-talk-joy-later-life-sex

19 Thunder, S., and Orsi, J., Song of the Deer: The Great Sundance Journey of the Soul (Jaguar Books, 1999), pp. 244–255

ABOUT THE AUTHOR

ITA O'BRIEN is one of the world's leading intimacy coordinators for film, TV, and theater and the creator of the Intimacy on Set Guidelines, which are now used around the world and have gained adoption in leading production houses, including HBO, Netflix, and the BBC. Ita, whose career spans over 40 years, has worked on a huge number of productions, including *Normal People, Conversations with Friends, I May Destroy You, It's a Sin, We Live in Time, Sex Education, Conversations with Friends, Dangerous Liaisons, Lady Chatterley's Lover, Empire of Light, Beetlejuice Beetlejuice, The Outrun,* and so many others.